TABLE OF CONTENTS

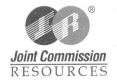

Joint Commission
RESOURCES

THE PHYSICIAN'S PROMISE

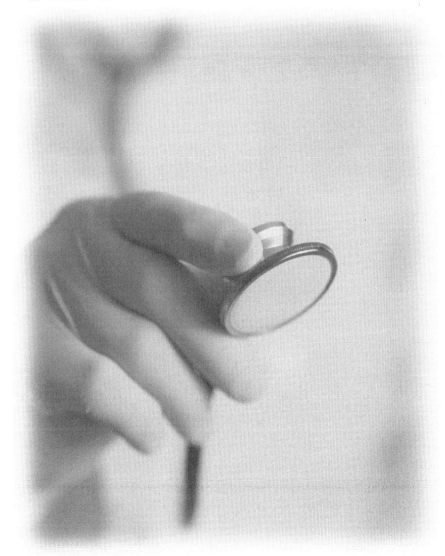

PROTECTING PATIENTS FROM HARM

Joint Commission Resources Mission

The mission of Joint Commission Resources is to continuously improve the safety and quality of care in the United States and in the international community through the provision of education and consultation services and international accreditation.

Joint Commission Resources educational programs and publications support, but are separate from, the accreditation activities of the Joint Commission. Attendees at Joint Commission Resources educational programs and purchasers of Joint Commission Resources publications receive no special consideration or treatment in, or confidential information about, the accreditation process.

FOREWORD

Problems in health care that lead to patient harm seldom have simple solutions. Accordingly, to arrive at meaningful solutions that will successfully prevent patient harm in the future, an all-encompassing systems-level approach to patient safety must be embraced in today's health care organizations—an approach that asks why an adverse event or close call occurred so as to prevent similar occurrences in the future.

The question "whose fault is it?" is inappropriate in that quest to understand why. The emphasis on prevention of harm must focus on learning, not punishment, to achieve meaningful, long-lasting improvement. This will not be easy, as a blame-seeking response has been ingrained in the medical profession over the years.

Einstein once defined insanity as doing the same thing over and over again and expecting different results. Health care professionals must be willing to look at health care systems differently than how we have in the past. Otherwise, we will continue to experience the same undesirable outcomes that we see in health care today.

The Physician's Promise: Protecting Patients from Harm provides many general and specific examples that illustrate strategies that can help in better understanding why patients are harmed and presents methods of preventing that harm. The topics covered in this book provide a tremendous opportunity for physicians to provide leadership in the much-needed enhancement of patient safety.

For the patient safety effort to be successful, it will require that physicians and the multidisciplinary teams with which they work learn new concepts and skills, many of which are extremely foreign to traditional medical training and are not presently part of our standard operating procedures.

Acquiring this knowledge is just the first step. To put that knowledge to use, physicians must practice using these techniques so that they not only become skillful in their application, but also are capable of providing leadership in their organizationwide adoption and implementation. Leadership is demonstrated through doing, not just talking.

Patient safety is not a finite goal that once achieved can be relegated to a lower priority. Patient safety can only be achieved through the relentless attention of those engaged in providing care to patients. It is a never ending journey, not a destination. This book is a tool that can be used to assist physicians on that journey.

James P. Bagian, MD, PE
Director, VA National Center for Patient Safety
November 2002

PREFACE

Purpose of the Publication

The Physician's Promise: Protecting Patients from Harm is written for physician leaders practicing in all health care settings and specialties. These leaders include physician chief executive officers (CEOs), directors of medical staffs, department heads, medical directors, physician deans, and all physicians who champion patient safety efforts in hospitals, ambulatory care facilities, critical access hospitals, physician offices, networks, laboratories, and assisted living, behavioral health, home care, and long term care organizations. This publication is also directed to those individuals, such as performance improvement, quality control, and risk managers, who work with physicians and other health care professionals in organizational settings to help monitor and improve safety and the quality of care and care outcomes.

The goal of *The Physician's Promise: Protecting Patients from Harm* is to further enhance the role assumed by physicians in the health care system to protect patients by preventing sentinel events.* At the culmination of their medical training, physicians embrace the Hippocratic Oath and/or other oaths and their role as advocate for those in their care. Contemporary medical practice most frequently

occurs through multidisciplinary teams in a complex environment characterized by dramatic technological and pharmacological advances and interdisciplinary care. Physicians therefore do not act alone. They serve in a leadership role, directing the creation of and follow-through on care plans. As such, their involvement in a leadership capacity is essential to the success of patient safety initiatives aimed at reducing sentinel events and improving the system failures at the root of these occurrences. Time and workload constraints make this particularly challenging for physicians.

This publication focuses on the role physicians play in protecting patients from harm in a team-based approach to patient care. The focus on physicians in no way implies that they are to blame for sentinel events or "near misses" that do occur, or that they are solely responsible for addressing patient safety challenges. Rather, this publication recognizes physicians' unique opportunity to proactively help identify and prevent systems-created failures.

Overview of Contents

The Physicians' Promise: Protecting Patients from Harm provides practical strategies physicians can use to identify and help prevent sentinel events. Each chapter identifies the specific type of sentinel event that physicians, working as leaders in a team-oriented environment, have the greatest potential to prevent. Sentinel event categories were identified by key stakeholders in the health care arena and Joint Commission on Accreditation of Healthcare Organizations (JCAHO) staff and surveyors trained

---

* A *sentinel event,* as defined by the Joint Commission on Accreditation of Healthcare Organizations, is an unexpected occurrence involving death or serious physical or psychological injury, or the risk thereof. The term *sentinel* is used because these events sound a warning that requires immediate attention. A sentinel event involves an unexpected variation in a process or an outcome that demands notice, understanding, and action.

in conducting analyses of system failures. JCAHO's sentinel event database and other nationally recognized studies on medical errors and health care safety provided needed data and analysis. A chapter-by-chapter description of the publication's contents follows.

An Introduction lays the groundwork, covering the state of medical failures in contemporary health care. The more informed perspective of errors views such adverse occurrences as the result of system failures rather than of individuals' negligence. An overview of key Institute of Medicine (IOM) studies examines the increased need in health care, as reported in these studies, to incorporate prevention strategies into the movement for identifying and reporting sentinel events. The introduction also describes major JCAHO patient safety initiatives and legislation and legal issues with an impact on patient safety.

Chapter 1: "The Role of Physicians in Today's Health Care Safety Environment" provides a brief historical look at the changing role of physicians in health care safety and describes in detail ways in which physician involvement in system analysis and error prevention activities can protect the patients in their care. The chapter outlines key proactive risk reduction activities, including improved communication, multidisciplinary team involvement, the use of technology, physician-generated care protocols or clinical practice guidelines, and education and training. A model for safety—initiatives in the field of anesthesiology—is described in order to provide readers with a sense of the range of possible solutions to safety challenges.

Six chapters then address how physicians can take a lead role in preventing specific types of sentinel events. Such events are those that physicians have the greatest potential to prevent because they are privy to relevant systems and processes that can and do fail: operative and postoperative errors and complications (Chapter 2); wrong-site, wrong-person, and wrong-procedure surgery (Chapter 3);

medication errors (Chapter 4); treatment delays with negative outcomes (Chapter 5); serious injury or death in physical restraints (Chapter 6); and suicide (Chapter 7).

Each of those six chapters includes an overview about why that particular sentinel event should be of concern to physicians, examples of near misses and sentinel events, the major system failures or root causes of such events, and practical strategies physicians can use to reduce the likelihood of their occurrence.

The examples of sentinel events and near misses included in this publication do not describe any actual event that has occurred in any specific organization. They are composites and adaptations of incidents that have occurred in numerous organizations and of those described in the professional literature. No example has been presented as it actually occurred. The Joint Commission vigorously protects the confidentiality of information learned during the accreditation process about sentinel events that have occurred in health care organizations and the root cause analyses of such events.

The "Selected Resources" chapter guides readers to articles, books, and reports on the topic of sentinel events and error reduction. The Appendix provides the Joint Commission's safety and error reduction standards, and the Index enables readers to access topics by key word.

A Note on Terminology and Requirements

Throughout the publication, the word *patient* is used to describe the individual person, client, consumer, or resident who actually receives health care and services. In addition, the authors try to minimize use of the word *error,* using *failure* instead whenever possible (see discussion in the Introduction). Specific Joint Commission requirements are outlined throughout the book. The proactive risk reduction strategies provided in each chapter are recommendations unless specifically stated as requirements tied to particular standards.

Acknowledgments

Thank you to Nancy Gorham Haiman for writing this publication. Her expertise is appreciated.

Thank you to Gregory J. Matz, MD, of Loyola University Medical Center in Maywood, Illinois for reviewing a portion of this publication. Many thanks also to the countless JCAHO and Joint Commission Resources staff members who contributed material to and reviewed this publication.

THE STATE OF MEDICAL FAILURES IN HEALTH CARE

Errors Versus System Failures

After decades of assigning individual blame for errors and "rooting out"—that is, firing, sanctioning, or reassigning—the "bad apples," health care leaders are starting to embrace the view of safety experts. These experts recognize that most errors are caused by system* problems or failures rather than by the individual negligence of physicians, nurses, or other health care professionals or providers. This represents a quantum shift in how leaders and their staff view problematic occurrences. In fact, it represents a step toward a new taxonomy for health care that redefines why "bad things"—for example, errors, failures, adverse occurrences, sentinel events, and so forth—happen.

In this new taxonomy, the term *error*† is being used less and less because it implies human involvement and fault. A *failure,* the term commonly used in other high-risk fields and increasingly used in health care instead of *error,* occurs because hazardous or latent conditions exist in systems or processes. *Latent conditions* are "pathogens" that are present within systems. They derive without intent from

decisions made (or not made) by system designers, top leaders, and others. Now frequently referred to as *hazardous conditions,* they often are overlooked. If detected, they can be corrected before they contribute to mishaps. If not addressed, these conditions can result in harm to individuals, but that harm is not always someone's fault or necessarily the result of human error.

The Beginning of a Transition

The health care world is transitioning from the old view of errors to the new view. The transition is neither synchronous nor universal, but, in the eyes of some, appears irrevocable.[2] The desire to assign individual blame for errors remains all too prevalent in contemporary health care. Because humans cannot possibly perform flawlessly, perfect performance is simply not a reasonable expectation. Doing the right thing right is the goal, but even when physicians and other health care professionals are focused exclusively on their work, working hard and working smart, things will go wrong. This way of thinking about errors represents a major shift from the entrenched zero-error-tolerance principles of traditional medicine.[3]

Commenting on the problem with the "First, do no harm," dictate, one writer observes:

> [I]t simply is not possible to do no harm all of the time. What's more, all practitioners know it. Virtually all drugs have adverse effects, many of them serious. Virtually all surgical procedures have an associated mortality and significant morbidity. Radiation and chemotherapy carry obvious harms.... Even simple bed rest predisposes to thromboembolic disease. Any intervention carries

---

* The definition of *system* according to the *Oxford American Dictionary of Current English* is "a set of connected things or parts." A more thorough definition is "any collection of components and the relationships between them, whether the components are human or not, when the components have been brought together for a well-defined goal or purpose."[1]

† JCAHO defines *error* as "the failure of a planned action to be completed as intended or the use of the wrong plan to achieve an aim."

Sidebar I-1. Examples of Problematic Systems That Elicit Human Errors

- Similar labeling on bottles; similar bottle shapes.
- Controls on equipment that do not operate as is customary and, hence, invoke different-than-expected actions.
- Lack of labeling on equipment connections that allows potentially lethal interconnections to be made.
- Operating room layout that requires wires to run across the floor in ways that make it likely that people will trip over them or accidentally pull them out of the socket.
- Noise levels in working environments that may cause messages to be misunderstood.
- Long work hours and extended shifts that increase the probability of individual error.

Source: Adapted from Moray N: Error reduction as a systems problem. In Bogner MS (ed): *Human Error in Medicine.* Hillsdale, NJ: Lawrence Erlbaum Associates, 1994, pp 68, 71. Used with permission.

risk. So any practitioner inevitably has patients who accrue harm as a result of his or her interventions. Furthermore, even doing nothing can result in harm… including failure to treat many conditions, failure to promote healthful behavior, and failure to heed the warning signs of a potentially suicidal patient. Even the wisest, most competent, most dedicated, and most careful among us makes mistakes.[3]

Award-winning physician and essayist Lewis Thomas notes that the ability to err represents the highest of human gifts. In his 1974 essay "To Err Is Human," he writes:

Mistakes are at the very base of human thoughts, embedded there, feeding the structure like root nodules. If we were not provided with the knack of being wrong, we could never get anything useful done. We think our way along by choosing between right and wrong alternatives, and the wrong choices have to be made as frequently as the right ones. We get along in life this way. We are built to make mistakes, coded for error…. The capacity to leap across mountains of information and land lightly on the wrong side represents the highest of human endowments.[4]

The New Outlook

Neville Moray of the University of Illinois at Urbana–Champaign sums up the new outlook on the relationship of errors to systems problems when he describes the perspective offered by human factors engineering pioneers Don Norman and James Reason: "[Their] fundamental claim is that the systems of which humans are a part call forth errors from humans, not the other way around. Only as an attribution of last resort, or because of the tendency of a legal system to be less concerned with justice than with economics, does one ascribe blame to an individual who commits an error."[1]

In a recent presentation titled "Creating a Culture of Safety," two experts describe what they call the "systems myth." This myth holds that there are two kinds of errors—human errors and systems errors—when, in reality, all errors are system errors. "Human errors are caused by system failures," they note.[5] There is always a systems answer to the question "Why?"

Sidebar I-1, left, provides a number of examples of how a system can elicit human errors.

The Role of Complexity

Health care is an exceedingly complex system. Accidents, errors, sentinel events, failures, and adverse events happen. Physicians and other practitioners working at the "sharp end" of the system must address competing demands, conflicts, and the expectation that their performance will be free of failure, while they interact with the hazardous processes demanded of their roles. Their patient care performance may be compromised by any number of common human factors, such as stress, fatigue, distractions, forgetfulness, haste, poor communication, and inaccurate assumptions. Meanwhile, those at the "blunt end" of the system—administrators, managers, insurance companies, suppliers—do not directly provide care, but they generate resources, constraints, and conflicts that produce latent conditions for those at the sharp end.[6] Failures occur. The challenges are to reduce the risk of failure, to protect patients from the failures that do occur, and, when failures do occur and reach the patient, to mitigate the effects of those failures on the patient.

Experts and organizations at the forefront of efforts to reduce medical errors recognize these failures as the symptoms of systems diseases. The diseases, not the symptoms, must be treated (that is, corrected or improved). Blaming an individual does not change the factors contributing to the failure. The failure is likely to recur. For example, one organization treated the *symptom* of a wrong-site surgery by revoking the clinical privileges of the physician who performed surgery on the incorrect site. Another organization treated the *disease* itself by developing and implementing a new multidisciplinary preoperative site verification process to prevent recurrence of the failure.

System components (for example, physicians, nurses, and other health care professionals), technological and pharmacological components (for example, computers, operating theaters, and drugs), management components (for example, policies and procedures), and financial components (for example, the reimbursement system that affects care decisions), must be designed properly and integrated into a cohesive, functioning whole.[1] Lasting change that reduces the future probability of failures is brought about only through systems improvement, not through the punishment of individuals. "Disciplinary treatment should be reserved for the unusual habitual rule-breakers, the 'cowboys,' who are not only dangerous, but also bad role models. Fortunately, these are rare," notes one expert.[7]

Spotlight on Health Care Safety

Released in 2000, the IOM's report *To Err Is Human: Building a Safer Health System*[8] catalyzed the professional and policymaking communities and the public at large around the critical issue of health care safety. The report indicates that at least 44,000 and perhaps as many as 98,000 Americans die each year as a result of medical errors.[8] Although not everyone agrees about the number of deaths resulting from medical errors, death attributed to this cause, even using IOM's lower estimate, constitutes one of the top ten causes of death in the United States. The report calls for a 50% reduction in the incidence of medical errors within five years.

Errors in the Public's Eye

Following highly publicized adverse events in 1994 and 1995 and the IOM report, public awareness of, and concern about, health care safety increased dramatically. Hospitals and other health care organizations appeared to be losing the confidence of the everyday citizen. According to a survey released in December 2000 by the Kaiser Family Foundation and the Agency for Healthcare Research and Quality (AHRQ), 47% of adults surveyed expressed serious doubts about obtaining error-free services in health care, in general, and, specifically, in hospitals.[9] This percentage is five points higher than data from a public opinion poll conducted for the National Patient Safety Foundation (NPSF) by Louis Harris & Associates, which found that 42% of adults surveyed believed that the current health care system does not have adequate measures in place to prevent medical mistakes.[10] The same percentage reported having been involved, either personally or through a friend or relative, in a situation where a medical mistake was made. More than two out of five had been involved in multiple situations. Respondents most frequently cited carelessness or negligence on the part of health care professionals as the main cause of medical mistakes. This reflects the pressing and widespread need to educate the public about the systems-based root of medical mistakes.

Individuals may always have felt some trepidation about the possibility of falling victim to medical error. However, with the release of the IOM report, it seemed that the public suddenly shifted from viewing incidents as unlikely anomalies to fearing that they are commonplace. This highlights perhaps the costliest aspect of medical error—the loss of trust in the health care system.

The Second IOM Report

On March 1, 2001, the IOM released its second report, *Crossing the Quality Chasm: A New Health System for the 21st Century.*[11] The report describes the U.S. health care system as "a tangled, highly fragmented web that often leaves unaccountable gaps in care and fails to build on the strengths of all health professionals."[12] It calls for immediate action to improve care and offers a comprehensive strategy to do so. Part of that strategy is monitoring and tracking by the U.S. Department of Health and Human Services of quality improvements in six key areas: safety, effectiveness, responsiveness, timeliness, efficiency, and equity. The report also offers ten rules intended, among other purposes, to promote the development of systems that are consciously and carefully designed to be safe, anticipate patient needs, promote cooperation among clinicians, use resources wisely, and make available information on quality and safety performance. According to the report, safety will be achieved and thus errors reduced not by asking health care workers to work harder but by fundamentally changing the way care is organized and delivered.

Need for Preventive Approach

The IOM reports, which built on the now classic Harvard Medical Practice Study,[13,14] and the NPSF's research on public opinion have cast a spotlight on the need to incorporate prevention strategies into the movement of identifying and reporting medical errors. The report of the Quality Interagency Coordination (QuIC) Task Force to the president, titled "Doing What Counts for Patient Safety: Federal Actions to Reduce Medical Errors and Their

Impact,"[15] brings this issue to the federal level by supporting the IOM's goal of reducing medical errors by 50% in five years. It also calls for administration efforts to improve the quality of health care by, among other initiatives, creating standards of health care safety. The Joint Commission is uniquely positioned for a leadership role in this function, as described in the next section.

Joint Commission Initiatives

The safety of health care has been an integral part of JCAHO's mission since the organization's inception. JCAHO has developed state-of-the-art, professionally based standards and evaluated the compliance of health care organizations and the professionals providing services under their aegis against these benchmarks since 1951. An analysis of current standards indicates that nearly 50% of JCAHO accreditation requirements relate to issues of health care safety. As JCAHO president Dennis S. O'Leary, MD, notes, this link is due to the fact that

[T]he accreditation process is, at its core, a risk reduction activity. It begins with the setting of contemporary standards that address important organization functions—for example, patient assessment, medication usage—and then encourages organizations, through the awarding of accreditation, to comply with these standards. The operating thesis is that if organizations are doing the "right things right," as reflected in the standards, then errors and adverse outcomes are less likely to happen than if there were no such standards. Notwithstanding the continued high frequency of errors, this thesis is almost certainly correct.[16]

In October 2002, the Joint Commission announced an initiative called "Shared Visions—New Pathways," picking up where Accreditation Process Improvement left off. The initiative aims to progressively sharpen the focus of the accreditation process on care systems that are critical to the safety and quality of patient care. Input from health care organizations and key stakeholders shaped the new accreditation process, which will provide a continuous picture of an organization's performance. The initiative includes, among other items, streamlined standards and a reduced documentation burden to focus more on critical patient care issues, a self-assessment process to support organizations' continuous standards compliance, and better engagement of physicians in the new accreditation process. The October 2002 issue of *Joint Commission Perspectives* (vol 22, no. 10) describes the new initiative in full.

The Role of Physicians

The Joint Commission believes that the active involvement of physicians in the accreditation process is critical—so much so that in 2002, JCAHO launched an initiative specifically to further engage physicians in JCAHO's accreditation process. The safety and quality of care provided in health care organizations depends on the entire organization as a system. Physicians are a critical component of the system. "The risk of errors in health care is high, an inevitable correlate of the intense human effort involved in patient care, the complexity of services provided, the expectations as a matter of public policy that care be provided with fewer resources, and the progressive introduction of new procedures, new technologies, and powerful new drugs, each with their potential great benefits and their potential for leading to patient harm," noted O'Leary during May 2002 congressional testimony.[17] Performance improvement in care quality and safety must be led jointly by the board, CEO, and medical staff.

As part of its Shared Visions—New Pathways initiative, JCAHO has implemented a strategic initiative to enhance the relevance of accreditation to physicians by better engaging them in the accreditation process and helping them provide safe and high-quality care. To achieve this objective, JCAHO has met with physicians who provide care in accredited and accreditable organizations. This dialogue focuses on patient safety, restraint use, pain management, and credentialing and other medical staff issues. In addition, the dialogue addresses JCAHO's desire to learn more about physician priorities and strategies for improving the quality and safety of care provided to their patients.

Information and Failure Reduction

The Joint Commission holds that information that guides the efforts of physicians, nurses, and other care professionals, and the managers that administer health care organizations is at the core of health care error reduction efforts. In testimony before House and Senate committees in February 2000, O'Leary outlined five critical information-based tasks whose completion is essential to an effective error reduction strategy:

1. Create a blame-free, protected environment that encourages the systematic surfacing and reporting of serious adverse events by physicians, nurses, and other health care professionals.
2. Produce credible "root cause" analyses of serious adverse events through the multidisciplinary involvement of physicians, nurses, administrators, and other members of the health care team.
3. Implement concrete, planned actions to reduce the likelihood of similar errors in the future through a multidisciplinary team process.
4. Establish safety standards that health care organizations must meet.
5. Disseminate experiential information learned from errors to all organizations at risk for serious adverse events.[18]

The Joint Commission addresses each of these tasks through its sentinel event policy and related activities, safety and health care error reduction standards, and new National Patient Safety Goals. These initiatives place the Joint Commission on the cutting edge of improving health care quality and safety and in a leadership position of addressing issues put forth in the IOM and subsequent reports.

JCAHO National Patient Safety Goals

In July 2002, JCAHO announced the first of the National Patient Safety Goals and Recommendations effective for all accreditation programs. For each of the goals, there are clear, evidence-based recommendations to help health care organizations reduce specific types of health care errors (see Sidebar I-2, page 7). Beginning January 1, 2003, the more than 17,000 JCAHO-accredited health care organizations that provide care relevant to the goals will be evaluated for compliance with the recommendations or implementation of acceptable alternative strategies. JCAHO expects to issue National Patient Safety Goals and Recommendations each year.

The 2003 goals were developed by an expert advisory group—the *Sentinel Event Alert* Advisory Group—composed of physicians, nurses, risk managers, and other professionals. The group reviewed the safety improvement recommendations in all published issues of *Sentinel Event Alert* for practicality, cost-effectiveness, and evidence base or expert consensus. "The goals and recommendations selected by the advisory group are all high-impact, low-cost targets," said Henri R. Manasse, Jr, PhD, chair of the *Sentinel Event Alert* Advisory Group, executive vice president and CEO of the American Society of Health-System Pharmacists, and past chair of the NPSF. "This initiative should really make a difference in improving patient safety."[19] The involvement of physicians and other health care professionals in implementation of the recommendations is critical.

Safety and Health Care Error Reduction Standards
JCAHO standards address a number of significant issues of direct interest to physicians and their patients. The Joint Commission has incorporated appropriate information learned from the analysis of sentinel events into accreditation standards. The JCAHO-approved standards directly focus on the safety of those receiving care and medical/health care error reduction. Implemented for hospitals effective July 2001, and for behavioral health care organizations effective January 2002, the initiative will extend to other programs in the next few years.

The standards were designed to improve health care safety and reduce risk to patients. They go beyond retrospective analysis of events to focus on proactively creating a culture of safety in health care organizations. They emphasize the proactive safety engineering of health care processes—using such techniques as failure mode and effects analysis—safety education of staff, and disclosure to the patient and family of significant unanticipated outcomes in care. Creating a proactive culture of safety depends on the active participation of physician leader champions.

Recognizing that effective medical/health care error reduction requires an integrated and coordinated approach, the standards relate specifically to leadership's role in an organizationwide safety program. This program includes all activities within the organization that contribute to the maintenance and improvement of health care safety, such as performance improvement, environmental safety, and risk management. The standards do not require the creation of new structures or offices within the organization; rather, they emphasize the need to integrate all care safety activities, both existing and newly created, with an identified focus of accountability within the organization's leadership, including medical staff leadership.

Effective reduction of medical/health care errors and other factors that contribute to unintended adverse health care outcomes in a health care organization requires an environment in which patients, their families, physicians, nurses, and other organization staff and leaders can identify and manage actual and potential risks to safety. This environment encourages recognition and acknowledgment of risks to patient safety and medical/health care errors. It also encourages the initiation of actions to reduce these risks and of the internal reporting of what has been found and the actions taken. The focus is on processes and systems. Individual blame or retribution for involvement in a medical/health care error is minimized. Organizational learning about medical/health care errors and sharing of that knowledge to effect behavioral changes in itself and in other health care organizations to improve the safety

Sidebar I-2. 2003 National Patient Safety Goals and Recommendations

Goal 1: Improve the accuracy of patient identification.
- Use at least two patient identifiers (neither to be the patient's room number) whenever taking blood samples or administering medications or blood products.
- Prior to the start of any surgical or invasive procedure, conduct a final verification process, such as a "time out," to confirm the correct patient, procedure, and site, using active–not passive–communication techniques.

Goal 2: Improve the effectiveness of communication among caregivers.
- Implement a process for taking verbal or telephone orders that requires a verification "read-back" of the complete order by the person receiving the order.
- Standardize the abbreviations, acronyms, and symbols used throughout the organization, including a list of abbreviations, acronyms, and symbols not to use.

Goal 3: Improve the safety of using high-alert medications.
- Remove concentrated electrolytes (including, but not limited to, potassium chloride, potassium phosphate, sodium chloride >0.9%) from patient care units.
- Standardize and limit the number of drug concentrations available in the organization.

Goal 4: Eliminate wrong-site, wrong-patient, and wrong-procedure surgery.
- Create and use a preoperative verification process, such as a checklist, to confirm that appropriate documents (for example, medical records, imaging studies) are available.
- Implement a process to mark the surgical site and involve the patient in the marking process.

Goal 5: Improve the safety of using infusion pumps.
- Ensure free-flow protection on all general-use and patient-controlled analgesia (PCA) intravenous infusion pumps used in the organization.

Goal 6: Improve the effectiveness of clinical alarm systems.
- Implement regular preventive maintenance and testing of alarm systems.
- Assure that alarms are activated with appropriate settings and are sufficiently audible with respect to distances and competing noise within the unit.

Source: Joint Commission: JCAHO approves National Patient Safety Goals for 2003. *Jt Comm Persp* 22(9):1–3, Sep 2002.

of those receiving care is pervasive. The leaders of the organization, including medical staff leaders, are responsible for fostering such an environment through their personal example and by establishing mechanisms that support effective responses to actual occurrences; through ongoing proactive reduction in medical/health care errors; and through integration of care safety priorities into the new design and redesign of all relevant organization processes, functions, and services.

A summary of major areas of focus in the safety standards follows:

- *Leadership:* Leaders create an environment that encourages error identification and remedial steps to reduce the likelihood of future, recurring errors.
- *Improving Organization Performance:* Health care organizations implement a program for proactive assessment of high-risk activities related to safety of patients and undertake appropriate improvements.
- *Management of Information:* Health care organizations aggregate safety-related data and information to identify risk to patients, apply knowledge-based information to reduce these risks, and promote effective communication among all caregivers and others involved in safety issues to guide and improve professional and organizational performance.
- *Rights:* The individual and/or the individual's family is informed about the outcomes of care, including unanticipated outcomes. Health care organizations are responsible for ensuring that the licensed independent practitioner (LIP)* or his or her designee clearly explains the outcome of any treatments or procedures to the individual and, when appropriate, the family, including those outcomes that differ significantly from the anticipated outcomes.
- *Other Functions:* Health care organizations place appropriate emphasis on safety in such areas as education of individuals and their families, continuity of care, and management of human resources.

Sentinel Event Program

Launched in 1996, the sentinel event program, including a sentinel event policy and the sentinel event database, emphasizes the requirement of root cause analysis for all sentinel events in accredited

---

* A *licensed independent practitioner* is any individual permitted by law and the hospital to provide care and services, without direction or supervision, within the scope of the individual's license and consistent with individually granted clinical responsibilities.

health care organizations. A detailed description of the sentinel event policy can be found in accreditation manuals and on the Joint Commission's Web site www.jcaho.org. Drawn from the sentinel event database, statistics on sentinel events reviewed by the Joint Commission since 1995 appear in Table I-1 page 9. These statistics are updated regularly on the JCAHO Web site.

To have a positive national effect on health care safety, information learned from errors—their occurrence, their characteristics, their effects or outcomes, and their root causes—must be aggregated, analyzed, and disseminated to the health care community at large. As part of the sentinel event policy, the Joint Commission disseminates information gleaned from errors and their root cause analyses to all organizations at risk for serious errors. In 1998 the Joint Commission began to periodically issue *Sentinel Event Alerts* to share with physicians, nurses, and other health care professionals the most important lessons learned from its database of sentinel events—known risks in systems and processes as well as safe practices. Newsletter topics appear in Sidebar I-3, page 10.

A New Taxonomy and Developing a Business Case for Patient Safety

Through an interorganizational workgroup, JCAHO is taking a leadership role in developing a patient safety taxonomy to be applied across all health care settings or domains. This will provide a common language with which national discussions on patient safety can continue unhindered by lack of agreement on definitions of key terms, such as *medical error*. The common language will allow organizations to collect and analyze patient safety data and disseminate safety information consistently.

According to the Joint Commission staff member who is spearheading the taxonomy effort, "The absence of a generally accepted patient safety taxonomy, or classification scheme, is one of the major barriers to a coordinated effort to improve safety. If we have a better understanding of errors through the use of a standardized patient safety taxonomy, we can use that information to mitigate the potential risk for errors and ultimately reduce the level of harm to patients."[20] He mentions that the taxonomy is intended to give the individual analyzing a medical failure a "big picture" of issues that should be investigated at the highest level. "It will be a tool for identifying different causative factors related to medical failures," he says.[21]

The taxonomy includes language describing the medical impact of a failure, such as "no harm" or "severe-permanent harm"; the *type* of failure, such as "communication," "patient management," and "clinical performance"; and the cause of the failure, such as "latent failures at the blunt end" (for example, training) and "active failures at the sharp end" (for example, failure in execution of preprogrammed and stored instructions or routine tasks). The goal is to increase understanding of the terms and their use without misinterpretation or misunderstanding among physicians, all other health care professionals and leaders, researchers, and the public.

In collaboration with the AHRQ, the Centers for Medicare and Medicaid Services (CMS), and the Department of Defense, JCAHO is striving to develop a business case for patient safety. Health care leaders commonly agree that making health care safer is an important priority. However, in the day-to-day world of hospitals and other health care organizations, investment in patient safety must compete for limited resources with other important initiatives. This joint initiative will demonstrate to CEOs and physician leaders of all health care organizations that efforts to improve patient safety are cost-effective. It will estimate the initial investment, maintenance, and payback for specific interventions and will identify the financial costs and potential savings associated with medical errors, standardization strategies (such as use of clinical practice guidelines), technological interventions, and infection control strategies, among others.

Table I-1. Sentinel Event Statistics

Type of Sentinel Event	Number	Percentage
Suicide	281	17.1%
Operative/Postop complications	200	12.2%
Medication error	190	11.5%
Wrong-site surgery	184	11.2%
Delay in treatment	87	5.3%
Falls	82	5.0%
Injury or death in restraints	78	4.6%
Assault/rape/homicide	69	4.2%
Transfusion error	43	2.6%
Perinatal loss of function/death	41	2.5%
Elopement	35	2.1%
Fire	32	1.9%
Ventilator injury/death	25	1.5%
Anesthesia-related event	24	1.5%
Medical equipment-related	24	1.6%
Infant abduction/release to wrong family	23	1.4%
Maternal death	20	1.2%
Death associated with transfer	14	0.9%
Other less frequent types	192	11.7%
Setting Where Event Occurred		
General hospital	1,031	62.6%
Psychiatric hospital	224	13.6%
Psych unit in general hospital	104	6.3%
Behavioral health care	93	5.7%
Long term care	63	3.8%
Emergency department	60	3.6%
Home care	36	2.2%
Ambulatory health care	29	1.8%
Clinical laboratory	5	0.3%
Health care network	1	0.1%

Since 1995, the Joint Commission has reviewed approximately 1,650 sentinel events. This table provides information on the types of sentinel events reviewed, their settings, sources for sentinel event identification, and sentinel event outcomes.

Or, lacking sufficient information to make a compelling business case for patient safety, the initiative will develop a research agenda to do so.

Other JCAHO initiatives in early stages of development include partnering with universities to create patient safety curricula for medical schools and developing public policy forums to address complex

Sidebar I-3.
Sentinel Event Alert Issues*

Bed Rail-Related Entrapment Deaths

Blood Transfusion Errors: Preventing Future
   Occurrences

Delays in Treatment

Exposure to Creutzfeldt-Jakob Disease

Fatal Falls: Lessons for the Future

High-Alert Medications and Patient Safety

Infant Abductions: Preventing Future Occurrences

Infusion Pumps: Preventing Future Adverse Events

Inpatient Suicides: Recommendations for
   Prevention

Kernicterus Threatens Healthy Newborns

Lessons Learned: Wrong Site Surgery

Lessons Learned: Fires in the Home Care Setting

Look-Alike, Sound-Alike Drug Names

Medical Gas Mix-ups

Medication Error Prevention—Potassium Chloride

Medication Errors Relating to Potentially
   Dangerous Abbreviations

Mix-up Leads to a Medication Error

Operative and Post-Operative Complications:
   Lessons for the Future

Preventing Needlestick and Sharps Injuries

Preventing Restraint Deaths

Preventing Ventilator-Related Deaths and Injuries

Wrong Site Surgery: A Follow-up Review

* Full *Sentinel Event Alert* issues can be accessed on the
   Joint Commission's Web site: www.jcaho.org. This list
   is complete as of the publication date.

patient safety issues, including staffing effectiveness, emergency preparedness, and emergency department (ED) overcrowding.

Error Disclosure: Requirements and New Legislation

The Joint Commission standard related to error disclosure requires that patients and, as appropriate, families be informed of the outcomes of care, including unanticipated outcomes. At a minimum, the patient and, when appropriate, the patient's

family must be informed about unanticipated outcomes of care that relate to sentinel events considered reviewable by the Joint Commission. The responsible LIP or his or her designee must inform the patient (and when appropriate, the patient's family) about these outcomes of care. These statements constitute the totality of Joint Commission requirements related to error disclosure. A discussion of legal and ethical duties Ito disclose and practical strategies for error disclosure as cited in the literature follow in this section. This information is offered not as Joint Commission requirements but rather as material illustrating what appears on error disclosure in the professional literature.

Errors Driven Underground

The still-prevalent punitive approach to errors— the desire to assign individual blame—drives errors underground in health care organizations. The myth of perfect performance creates feelings of emotional distress and inadequacy in anyone making a mistake. If the physician's or other health care professional's mistake causes harm, then guilt and remorse often predominate. In researcher Albert Wu's words, "Although patients are the first and obvious victims of medical mistakes, doctors are wounded by the same errors: they are the second victims."[22]

The pressure to be perfect provides strong incentive to cover up mistakes rather than disclose them and address underlying root causes. Organizations as well as individuals may hide or refuse to discuss an error, exhibiting behavior described by one expert as "circling the wagon" in a protective silence.[23] Such an approach to errors must change in health care in order to provide lasting change and to protect individuals receiving care from harm. Wu describes how a practitioner feels after making a mistake: "You feel singled out and exposed—seized by the instinct to see if anyone has noticed. You agonize about what to do, whether to tell anyone, what to say…. You question your competence but fear being discovered. You know you should confess, but dread the prospect of potential punishment and the patient's anger."[22] He notes a lack of appropriate forums for physicians' discussion of errors.

Legal Duty to Disclose

Physicians' legal duty to disclose medical errors is clear and stems from case law. Courts have ruled that physicians are required to disclose all pertinent information to patients due to the fiduciary nature of the physician–patient relationship.

Ethical Duty to Disclose

Notwithstanding legal obligations, disclosure of medical errors by physicians has long been recognized by the medical profession as an ethical responsibility. Disclosure is simply "the right thing to do." It is a physician's responsibility as a professional and an advocate for patients in his or her care and part of his or her "promise."

Ethical requirements published by major medical organizations address the need for physicians to disclose errors with significant consequence, but the requirements are less clear on the disclosure of minor events.[24] The American Medical Association's (AMA's) *Code of Medical Ethics: Current Opinions with Annotations* states:

> Situations occasionally occur in which a patient suffers significant medical complications that may have resulted from the physician's mistake or judgment. In these situations, the physician is ethically required to inform the patient of all the facts necessary to ensure understanding of what has occurred. Only through full disclosure is a patient able to make informed decisions regarding future medical care.... Concern regarding legal liability, which might result following truthful disclosure, should not affect the physician's honesty with a patient.[25]

The American College of Physicians *Ethics Manual,* 4th Edition, states: "Physicians should disclose to patients information about procedural and judgment errors made in the course of care, if such information is material to the patient's well-being. Errors do not necessarily constitute improper, negligent, or unethical behavior, but failure to disclose them may."[26]

Disclosure and Trust

Beyond the ethical issue is the practical issue of trust. Patients simply expect their physician to disclose errors made during treatment, even minor errors. "Because trust is a fundamental ingredient of the patient–physician relationship, and trust is dependent in part on communication and truth telling, that trust is diminished by secrecy, hiding, or misleading information," notes Paul M. Schyve, MD, senior vice president of the Joint Commission.[27] One study indicates that 98% of patients expected their physician to acknowledge an error, regardless of its severity, and were more likely to consider litigation if the physician did not disclose the error.[28]

Reluctance to Disclose

Good physician–patient communication is instrumental in achieving positive care outcomes. Yet health care professionals often do not tell patients or families about their mistakes. Only 24% of house officers anonymously surveyed in a now-classic study by Wu and his colleagues told the patient or family of their errors in diagnosis, prescription, evaluation, communication, and procedural complications that led to serious outcomes in 90% of the cases, including death in 31%.[29] Fear of malpractice litigation, the threat of professional sanctions, and the myth of perfect performance discussed earlier reinforce poor provider communication of errors to patients.

A 1999 study provides supporting data. Only 60% of physicians participating in the survey believed that a patient should *always* be told if a complication has occurred, while 92% of patients thought they should be told of adverse events.[30] "[A] doctor's reluctance to provide detailed information to patients after adverse events is often an attempt to protect the patient from potentially detrimental anxiety. However, doctors may also avoid telling patients because it is a time consuming, difficult, and unpleasant task and because they fear losing a patient's trust, being blamed, and perhaps being sued," writes the study's lead author.[30]

Disclosure and Malpractice Suits

The current malpractice environment is frequently cited as a deterrent to the disclosure and openness required for performance improvement.[31] Paradoxically, research studies suggest that physician openness and full disclosure *reduce* the likelihood of law suits. One survey conducted at Loma Linda University found that 41% of victims of medical errors who filed malpractice suits said there *was* something that could have been done that would have reduced their need to take legal action. Of these, 37% said that they would not have sued if they had received an explanation and an apology.[32]

Data from a study conducted at the Veterans Affairs Medical Center in Lexington, Kentucky, are equally encouraging.[33] Following two costly unsuccessful defenses of malpractice cases, that organization instituted a proactive policy for the following:
- Early review of patient injuries caused by accidents or negligence that could result in litigation;
- Full disclosure of findings to the patient;
- Assistance to the family with filing any necessary claims forms; and
- Fair compensation.

Unexpectedly, the policy did not cause an onslaught of litigation, and, overall, the organization realized a cost savings, due in part to lower legal expenses.[34] One expert summarizes, "Full disclosure of errors and just compensation for injuries seems to be an ethical, cost-effective solution. It restores organizations and practitioners to a patient advocacy role, putting the patient's interests first, while potentially minimizing the organization's financial impact. It encourages open communication about errors and helps restore the public's trust in health care. It's the right thing to do."[35]

The Hows of Disclosure

Communication and disclosure involve more than notification of the patient. Communication by the provider with all relevant parties following the occurrence of a sentinel event or mistake that led or could have led to patient injury is critical. In addition to the patient and family, relevant parties include
- colleagues who could provide support and gain the opportunity to learn from the error;
- the health care organization's and provider's liability insurers;
- appropriate organizational staff, including risk managers or quality assurance representatives; and
- others who could provide emotional support or problem-solving help for the individual who made the error.

Disclosing mistakes to patients and their families is difficult, at best. Yet many legal and ethical experts generally advise practitioners to disclose mistakes to patients and/or their families in as open, honest, and forthright a manner as possible. Wu and colleagues suggest that disclosure of a mistake may foster learning by compelling the physician to acknowledge the error truthfully.[36] Sidebar I-4, pages 13–14, presents the procedure for disclosure of medical accidents developed and distributed by the Minnesota Hospital and Healthcare Partnership, a coalition of Minnesota's health care community.

The Confidentiality of Disclosure

The confidentiality of apologies and peer review data related to medical errors is a major issue for health care organizations and professionals. A few states have enacted laws supporting the inadmissibility in malpractice cases of physicians' expressions of sympathy. Courts in a handful of states have similarly protected the confidentiality of physicians' apologies. Troyen A. Brennan, lead researcher of the landmark Harvard Medical Practice Study, describes the need to reform the malpractice litigation system: "Any effort to prevent injury due to medical care is complicated by the dead weight of a litigation system that induces

Sidebar I-4. Procedure for Disclosure of Medical Accidents

Patients or the appropriate guardian or representative have the right to a prompt and truthful conversation when a medical accident occurred.

To assure continuity and appropriate perspective in discussion, the disclosure of information and subsequent discussions with the patient or his/her guardian or representative will be handled by the responsible licensed independent practitioner or his/her designee. In most cases, the licensed practitioner caring for the patient is the preferred communicator in the disclosure of unanticipated outcomes.

Organizations may wish to have the practitioner inform appropriate administrative personnel before discussing such outcomes with the patient for the purposes of mentoring the individual on how to handle the discussion, reviewing what should be discussed, and the initiation of the organization's support, risk management, and quality assurance functions as may be required.

Consideration should be given to having a second individual present during the initial conversation with the patient or the appropriate guardian or representative of the patient to assist with documentation of the conversation and to provide continuity and clarity.

Facts will be reviewed and shared with the patient or appropriate guardian or representative without unnecessary delay.

In rare instances where disclosure of a medical accident will have a deleterious effect on the patient's well being, disclosure may be withheld until such a time that the benefits of disclosure are greater than the harm.

For discussions anticipated to be complex or difficult, patients or appropriate guardians or representatives should be given the option of having another person with them as support during the discussion.

During initial and follow-up discussion the following subjects may be discussed, although discussion of each subject on the list is not required nor is discussion limited to these topics:

- The hospital and its staff regret and apologize that a medical accident has occurred.
- The nature of the medical accident.
- The time, place, and circumstances of the medical accident.
- The proximate cause of the medical accident, if known.
- The known, definite consequences of the medical accident for the patient and potential consequences.
- Actions taken to treat or ameliorate the consequences of the medical accident.
- Who will manage ongoing care of the patient.
- Planned investigation or review of the medical accident.
- Who else has been informed of the medical accident (in the hospital, review organizations, etc.) and the facility's confidentiality policy.
- Actions taken to identify systems issues that may have contributed to the medical accident and to prevent the same or similar medical accident from reoccurring.
- Who will manage ongoing communication with the patient or appropriate guardian or representative.
- The names and phone numbers of individuals in the hospital to whom the patient or appropriate guardian or representative may address complaints or concerns about the process around the medical accident.

(continued)

Sidebar I-4. Procedure for Disclosure of Medical Accidents (continued)

- The names and phone numbers of agencies to whom the patient or appropriate guardian or representative could communicate about the medical accident.
- How to obtain support and counseling regarding the medical accident and its consequences both within the hospital and from outside.
- The organization's process to establish compensation for harm, as appropriate— or contact person's name.

The facts and pertinent points of the conversation with the patient and/or family will be recorded in the medical record.

Appropriate communications are made internally within the health care facility and are consistent with organizational practices such as public relations, risk management, and media policies.

Source: Excerpted from *Communicating Outcomes to Patients.* (brochure). Minnesota Hospital and Healthcare Partnership, St Paul, MN, 2002. Used with permission.

secrecy and silence. No matter how much we might insist that physicians have an ethical duty to report injuries resulting from medical care or to work on their prevention, fear of malpractice litigation drags us back to the status quo."[37]

Legislation introduced in the U.S. Senate in June 2002 by Senators Jeffords, Frist, Breaux, and Gregg—the Patient Safety and Quality Improvement Act—would encourage the voluntary reporting of health care errors by protecting the confidentiality of reports of serious adverse events and the analyses of underlying causes (root cause analyses). Federal peer review protections would be granted for information related to medical errors reported by medical professionals to a certified patient safety organization. "Removing the fear of lawsuits is key to enticing more physicians and hospitals to come forward voluntarily with information about patient safety," says Senator Jeffords. "If you don't get the information, you can't address the problems."[38]

JCAHO, which has been encouraging such legislation for years, lauded the bill as a breakthrough in the blame-and-punishment orientation of current society.[39] JCAHO, the AMA, the IOM, and other organizations maintain that because there is so much uncertainty about the confidentiality of error-related information, errors continue to be driven underground, thereby impeding patient safety improvements. The bill affords some measure of hope about the possibility of a permanent fix for this national problem.

Concluding Comments

The recognition of sentinel events or medical failures as system failures rather than the mistakes of individuals does not preclude the important role the individual physician can play in identifying the potential for sentinel events and preventing them, where possible. The key systems issues most frequently cited to be at the root of sentinel events involve staffing, training, communication, and culture. These represent the greatest challenge to the provision of safe care by all health care professionals. Chapter 1 describes the role of physicians in today's health care safety environment and four proactive approaches physicians can consider as fundamental to their overall efforts to protect patients from harm.

REFERENCES

1. Moray N: Error reduction as a systems problem. In Bogner MS (ed): *Human Error in Medicine.* Hillsdale, NJ: Lawrence Erlbaum Associates, 1994, p 71.
2. Cook RI: Two years before the mast: Learning how to learn about patient safety. Presented at Enhancing Patient Safety and Reducing Errors in Health Care (Annenberg II), Rancho Mirage, CA, 8–10 Nov 1998.

3. Shelton JD: The harm of "First, do no harm." *JAMA* 284:2687–8, 6 Dec 2000.

4. Thomas L: *The Medusa and the Snail: More Notes of a Biology Writer.* New York: Viking Press, 1974, pp 37–9.

5. Jones FG, Hallman C: Creating a culture of safety. Presented at CSR Orion II, Atlanta, Jan 2002.

6. Cook RI: A brief look at the new look on complex system failure, error, and safety. Cognitive Technologies Laboratory (unpublished paper), 2001.

7. Spencer FC: Human error in hospitals and industrial accidents: Current concepts. *J Am Coll Surg* 191:410–8, Oct 2000.

8. Institute of Medicine: *To Err Is Human: Building a Safer Health System.* Washington, DC: National Academy Press, 2000.

9. Kaiser Family Foundation (KFF) and the Agency for Healthcare Research and Quality: *National Survey on Americans as Health Care Consumers: An Update on the Role of Quality Information.* Menlo Park, CA: KFF, 2000. Web site: www.kff.org.

10. National Patient Safety Foundation at the American Medical Association: *Public Opinion of Patient Safety Issues: Research Findings.* Chicago Sep 1997. Web site: www.npsf.org.

11. Institute of Medicine: *Crossing the Quality Chasm: A New Health System for the 21st Century.* Washington, DC: National Academy Press, 2001.

12. National Academy of Sciences: U.S. health care delivery system needs major overhaul to improve quality and safety (press release). Washington, DC, 1 Mar 2001. Web site: www4.nationalacademies.org/news.nsf/isbn/0309072808.

13. Brennan TA, et al: Incidence of adverse events and negligence in hospitalized patients: Results of the Harvard Medical Practice Study I. *NEJM* 324:370–76, 7 Feb 1991.

14. Leape LL, et al: The nature of adverse events in hospitalized patients: Results of the Harvard Medical Practice Study II. *NEJM* 324:377–84, 7 Feb 1991.

15. Quality Interagency Coordination Task Force: *Doing what counts for patient safety: Federal actions to reduce medical errors and their impact.* Report to the President, Feb 2000. Web site: www.quic.gov.

16. O'Leary DS: Editorial: Accreditation's role in reducing medical errors. *BMJ* 320:727–8, Mar 2000.

17. O'Leary DS: Statement of the Joint Commission on Accreditation of Healthcare Organizations before the House Committee on Energy and Commerce Subcommittee on Health, 8 May 2002.

18. O'Leary DS: Statement of the Joint Commission on Accreditation of Healthcare Organizations before the Committee on Health, Education, Labor and Pensions, U.S. Senate and the Subcommittee on Labor, Health and Human Services, and Education of the Senate Committee on Appropriations, 22 Feb 2000.

19. As quoted in Joint Commission on Accreditation of Healthcare Organizations: Joint Commission announces National Patient Safety Goals (press release), 24 Jul 2002.

20. Joint Commission: Patient safety taxonomy: One step to reducing errors. *Jt Comm Persp on Patient Safety* 2:1, 3, Aug 2002.

21. Personal communication with Andrew Chang, JD, MPH, 22 Aug 2002.

22. Wu AW: Medical error: The second victim: The doctors who makes the mistake needs help too. *BMJ* 320:726–7, 18 Mar 2000.

23. Darr K: Uncircling the wagons: Informing patients about unanticipated outcomes. *Hosp Topics* 79:33–5, summer 2001.

24. Rosner F, et al: Disclosure and prevention of medical errors. *Arch Intern Med* 160:2089–92, 24 Jul 2000.

25. American Medical Association (AMA) Council on Ethical and Judicial Affairs: *Code of Medical Ethics: Current Opinions with Annotations,* 1996–1997 Edition. Chicago: AMA, 1997, sect 8.12:125.

26. American College of Physicians: *Ethics Manual,* 4th ed. Reprinted in *Ann Intern Med* 128:576–94, 1998.

27. Personal communication with Paul M. Schyve, MD, Jul 2002.

28. Witman AB, Park DM, Hardin SB: How do patients want physicians to handle mistakes? A survey of internal medicine patients in an academic setting. *Arch Intern Med* 156:2565–9, 9–23 Dec 1996.

29. Wu AW, et al: Do house officers learn from their mistakes? *JAMA* 265(16):2089–94, 1991.

30. Hingorani M, Wong T, Vafidis G: Patients' and doctors' attitudes to amount of information given after unintended injury during treatment: Cross sectional, questionnaire survey. *BMJ* 318:640–1, 6 Mar 1999.

31. Blumenthal D: Making medical errors into medical treasures. *JAMA* 272(23):1851–7, 1994.

32. Vincent CA, et al: Why do people sue doctors? A study of patients and relatives taking legal action. *Lancet* 343:1609–13, 25 Jun 1994.

33. Kraman SS, Hamm G: Risk management: Extreme honesty may be the best policy. *Ann Intern Med* 131:963–7, 21 Dec 1999.

34. Wu AW: Handling hospital errors: Is disclosure the best defense? *Ann Intern Med* 131:970–2, 21 Dec 1999.

35. Smetzer J: Prescriptions for safety. *AHA News,* 20 Mar 2000.

36. Wu AW, et al: To tell the truth: Ethical and practical issues in disclosing medical mistakes to patients. *J Gen Int Med* 12:770–5, Dec 1997.

37. Brennan TA: The Institute of Medicine Report on medical errors—Could it do harm? *NEJM* 342:1123–5, 13 Apr 2000.

38. As quoted in Landa AS: Patient safety bill calls for voluntary error reporting. *AMNews* 45(25): 1 Jul 2002.

39. Joint Commission: Joint Commission commends Patient Safety and Quality Improvement Act (press release). Oakbrook Terrace, IL, 7 Jun 2002.

CHAPTER 1

THE ROLE OF PHYSICIANS IN TODAY'S HEALTH CARE SAFETY ENVIRONMENT

A Brief Look into History

Not too long ago, the vast majority of health care in the United States was provided by a lone physician who traveled to the patient's home, armed with a little—or perhaps not so little—black bag. This replaced the system of care prevalent in Colonial America, which involved care of the sick and injured by family members and mutual assistance provided by lay community members. In his book titled *The Social Transformation of American Medicine,* Paul Starr describes: "[A]s larger towns and cities grew [during the late nineteenth century], treatment increasingly shifted from the family and lay community to paid practitioners, druggists, hospitals, and other commercial and professional sources."[1] The physician of the late nineteenth and early twentieth century was usually an autonomous decision maker whose scientifically based knowledge was increasingly valued by society.

As the pace of technological advances quickened in the twentieth century, care provided by physicians for the acutely ill or injured increasingly shifted from homes or community-based offices to the hospital setting. The newly emerging emergency medical service providers responded to calls from homes and picked up patients for transport to hospitals. Physicians continued to direct the patient's care in the hospital but generally remained independent of the hospitals' organizational structure.[1] This often created tension between organizational and practitioner objectives. Both desired high-quality care outcomes, but, due to time constraints, physicians increasingly resisted the information requirements "imposed" by hospitals in such areas as credentialing, clinical records, and continuing professional education.

Meanwhile, technological advances also enabled much non-acute care to be provided in ambulatory settings. During the 1970s and 1980s, office-based surgery and diagnostics began to flourish as physicians increasingly provided non-acute care in outpatient settings. Simultaneously, reimbursement constraints resulting from ever-rising health care costs forced hospitals and physicians to discharge hospitalized patients to home care, postacute, or long term care settings earlier and in a more acute or unstable condition. This affected physicians' ability to monitor patients' health postdischarge.

Current Leadership Role in Health Care Safety

Today, physicians maintain their leadership role in patient care, but the environment in which they work and the role they play in that environment have changed. Highly complex and advanced, health care now is an interdisciplinary process. With physicians serving as leaders, health care systems and processes involve teams of professionals practicing in a variety of organizational settings. Care is collaborative. This means that ensuring the safety of individuals receiving care also must be collaborative.

As advocates for the individuals in their care, physicians are in a leadership position with respect to improving health care safety. "Physicians have traditionally asked themselves what they can do better to improve their patients' outcomes. More recently, we are hearing physicians ask what they can do to prevent harm to their patients," says Paul Schyve, MD, JCAHO senior vice president.[2] "That is why it is important for physicians to think about how the system in which they work should be improved."

Physicians are accustomed to thinking about systems—physiological systems. When they search for the cause of an individual's symptoms, they look for pathology in the various systems of the human body. All too often, however, there may be a reluctance to apply this mode of thinking to the social and technical context of the health care organization. Physicians need to think about health care systems because they work within the systems and their work is compromised by failures and problems within these. For example, laboratory reports and nursing charts are vital to physician decision making. Reports or charts that are misread or attached to the wrong patient represent an information management system failure. Physicians must provide input into the information management system to make sure that it meets their needs and those of their patients and assures that failures do not compromise patient safety.

"Physicians must be involved in performance improvement efforts to improve the core of what a health care organization is all about—providing quality health care," says Schyve.[2] Improving health care safety through systems improvement must be viewed by physicians not as an "extra" activity but as a driving force of the profession. Physician champions must bring this issue forward, and the profession must build it into continuing professional development.

As the complexity of health care increases, so too does the need to monitor and prevent medical system failures. In earlier decades, physicians were responsible chiefly for responding to errors. In this decade, physicians at the grassroots level must assume a leadership role in proactive risk reduction. Forums for discussing sentinel events and how to

reduce the likelihood of their occurrence with colleagues, other health care professionals, risk managers, and organization leaders must be created. "Caregivers need to understand the issues and know that they are not the problem but instead are part of the solution," note two authors.[3] Patients and their families must also be involved in safety-related conversations and forums. The Joint Commission's "Speak Up" initiative is designed to increase patient involvement and communication with caregivers in order to reduce medical failures. Brochures distributed to health care organizations, physician offices, and pharmacies and buttons bearing the Speak Up slogan encourage patients and families to inform caregivers if they have questions or concerns about some aspect of care.

Anesthesiology: A Model for Health Care Safety

Much can be learned about developing a preventive approach to protecting patients from harm by examining the now decades-old initiatives in the field of anesthesiology. Anesthesiology led the way among medical specialties in identifying patient safety issues and pioneering systems-oriented solutions. Lucian Leape and his colleagues write, "Anesthesia is the only system in health care that begins to approach the vaunted 'six sigma' level of perfection that other industries strive for. Mortality from elective anesthesia has declined 10-fold in the past several decades as the result of a concerted effort to improve safety."[4] Anesthesiology was the first to establish practice standards and was also the first to establish a private patient safety foundation. The Anesthesia Patient Safety Foundation (APSF), founded in 1985, in fact, was used as the model for the NPSF, founded by the AMA in 1998.

Why the field of anesthesiology? Accidents due to errors in anesthesiology can be dramatic, resulting in death or serious brain injury to patients. Early data indicated that in spite of careful preoperative evaluation and planning, nearly 20% of anesthesia cases involved unanticipated problems that could harm the patient and that required intervention by the anesthesiologist.[5] Some 3% to 5% of cases involved serious unplanned events that required substantial intervention, with or without full recovery of the patient.[6]

One expert describes operating rooms (ORs), the environment in which anesthesiologists practice, as "hotbeds for human error."[7] They are complex and dynamic, with constant change and time pressures. High-technology equipment is used extensively, as are potentially lethal drugs. Situational or environmental factors, including long working hours, boredom, and intensive technology, impinge on human performance. Procedures require the effort of physicians and nurses working smoothly as a team. An anesthesiologist works with severe time pressures and within a tightly coupled system that provides no opportunity for recovery. *Tightly coupled* processes or systems have steps that follow one another in such rapid sequence that a variation occurring in one step cannot be responded to before the next step occurs. A failure of one step can lead to a "cascade of failure" as each following step tries to handle an input it was not designed to handle and fails as a result. Failures frequently occur at the point where one process or step overlaps or "hands off" to another.

The study of human error in anesthesiology commenced comparatively early, catalyzed by the malpractice crisis of the 1970s. Jeffrey Cooper and his colleagues at Massachusetts General Hospital were among the first to study critical incidents in medicine.[8] David Gaba and his colleagues analyzed the chain of evolution of sentinel events during anesthesia, identifying proximate causes* and underlying latent errors.[9] Strong leaders who, according to Gaba, "were willing to admit that patient safety was imperfect and that, like any other medical problem, patient safety could be studied and

interventions planned to achieve better outcomes" emerged to champion the patient safety effort.[10]

The results have been dramatic. In the early 1980s anesthesia mortality was approximately 2 deaths per 10,000 anesthetics administered. Today, the rate is 1 death per 200,000 to 300,000 anesthetics. Preventive failure reduction strategies used in the field of anesthesiology to achieve these impressive results cluster into four distinct categories: technological solutions, standards and guidelines, education and training, and collaborative teamwork. A description of each follows.

Technological Solutions

In the realm of *technological solutions,* electronic monitoring has contributed significantly to improved patient safety.[11] Monitors and alarms introduced on anesthesia equipment are now highly effective in helping the anesthesia team prevent negative outcomes. In the late 1980s John Tinker and colleagues at the University of Iowa reported the results of a large study evaluating the preventive benefits of two monitoring technologies—pulse oximetry and capnometry.[12] Applied together, the two technologies were considered potentially preventive in 93% of the preventable anesthetic mishaps.

Also on the equipment front, in the mid-1980s, breaking circuit disconnection was the most frequent critical incident leading to serious adverse outcomes. Engineered safety devices were introduced to physically prevent errors from being made. Gaba cites the classic example of such a device—the system of gas connectors that prevent a gas hose or cylinder from being installed at the wrong site.[10] Such fail-safe design provides an effective barrier that allows intervention in some way, either through humans or through an automated response to protect the individual receiving care. New devices to manage patients' airways and new display technologies to minimize errors and maximize data transfer during complex patient care are other examples of technological solutions to reduce the likelihood of sentinel events.

---

* *Proximate causes* are the superficial, obvious, or immediate causes of a sentinel event.

Standards and Guidelines

Anesthesiologists adopted *standards and guidelines* as an effective error reduction strategy as early as the 1980s. These clinical guidelines or practice parameters covered the diagnosis, management, and treatment of various problems frequently encountered by the anesthesiologist. Standards included electrocardiographic monitoring, assessment of ventilation, use of pulse oximetry, and use of capnography to measure carbon dioxide levels during general anesthesia.[10]

Diagnostic and corrective protocols have been developed based on studies identifying the need for protocols for preoperative assessment of patients, for preoperative inspection of equipment and apparatus, and for the exchange of anesthesia personnel. The failure to detect machine leaks, the failure to review patient records leading to complications from a contraindicated drug, the failure to have needed drugs on an anesthesia tray before a crisis, and the failure to review the patient's medical status when one anesthesiologist replaced another were all cited as incidents that could have been prevented through the use of protocols.[13] Guidelines and criteria for determining whether to proceed with surgery reduce production pressures frequently encountered by anesthesiologists.

Education and Training

Anesthesiology has been at the forefront of the medical profession in *training and educational* efforts aimed at reducing medical failures. This specialty pioneered the use of complete environment-realistic simulators and computer screen simulators to evaluate decision making and performance of trainees and practitioners. Anesthesiologist trainees and practitioners use simulators, based on those used by airline pilots, to learn how to manage critical incidents. The patient, monitors, and management choices are displayed via a computer program. Simulator users act out various roles, employing an electronically controlled dummy attached to real monitors that simulate patient conditions and

reactions. Data based on simulator studies have been used to identify and act on improvement opportunities. Experience and practice in reacting to intraoperative problems have been shown to be significant factors in the speed of appropriate correction of the simulated problems, leading to recommendations for increased simulator-based training.[14]

Anesthesiology has long emphasized the importance of continuing professional education. For example, early on, the American Society of Anesthesiology took a proactive role in evaluating anesthetic complications in order to share the information learned with practicing anesthesiologists. The Tinker study described earlier involved the review by physician anesthesiologists of approximately 1,200 closed malpractice claims against anesthesiologists provided by 17 professional liability insurers. Its results were broadly disseminated and developed into best practices recommendations.[12]

Teamwork

The effectiveness of individuals working as a team in reducing and preventing errors has been studied in great depth in the field of anesthesiology. The field has fully embraced *a collaborative, team approach*. Team-enhancing exercises, such as Crew Resource Management (CRM), is used extensively in anesthesiology to alleviate communication failures such as those that occur when anesthesiologists do not interrupt or contradict surgeons or when nurse anesthetists or residents fail to call their supervisors or speak up on issues that affect patient safety.

CRM originated and is used extensively in the airline industry as a tool to improve performance with flight, cabin, ground, and maintenance crews. Its success in increasing morale, teamwork, coordination, and communication to reduce and prevent errors has been significant. The CRM technique views crews as a resource for solving problems and gives such crews experience via simulation, role playing, and other strategies in handling crisis situations. Humans are *the* critical resource in dealing with novel, threatening situations. CRM training includes, among other things, self-critique, communication skills, personality assessments, distraction avoidance, interpersonal relationships, leadership–followership issues, and overall technical proficiency and crew effectiveness.

Like airline crews, medical professionals working in OR and ED settings and those coordinating the services of many departments and disciplines in ordinary patient care units are highly technically trained, must respond quickly in emergencies, work within a task-interdependent environment, and participate in teams whose composition changes frequently. Smoothly functioning teamwork is critical to patient safety.

Although the contributions from anesthesiology of each of the four failure-reduction strategies described above have been enormous, Gaba writes, "In the long term the most important contribution of anaesthesiology to patient safety may be the institutionalization and legitimization of patient safety as a topic of professional concern."[10] Indeed, capturing physician interest in and commitment to patient safety as a part of their continuing professional development is vital to improved patient care.

Physician involvement in efforts to enhance the safety of individuals in their care can, as in anesthesiology, focus on the following areas: education and training, care protocols or clinical practice guidelines, technological solutions, and collaborative teamwork and improved communication. A current description of the "state of the art" for each follows.

Proactive Approach 1: Education and Training
The Need for Focus
Health care organizations that completed root cause analyses of sentinel events in their facilities identified insufficient orientation/training as a root cause of 58% of reviewed events and competency/credentialing as a root cause of 12% of reviewed

events. Education and training provide the foundation of professional competence and constitute both traditional proactive and reactive initiatives to reduce and prevent failures.

Traditional Medical Education
Medical education in the United States has traditionally emphasized the teaching of a core of knowledge focused largely on the basic mechanisms of disease and pathophysiological principles.[15] The Flexner Report of 1910 outlines the key structure of medical school curriculum at that time. The curriculum involved two years of basic sciences and two years of clinical training. Once trained in basic principles, physicians were granted moral autonomy and expected to learn from their mistakes, for the most part, answerable to themselves only.[16]

One writer describes the perception of physicians prevalent in the early 1900s as authoritative agents whose "character, rather than empirical standards, provided the basis for evaluation," and notes, "this model of accountability contributed nothing to general knowledge about therapeutic safety or effectiveness, why mistakes might occur, or how they could be prevented."[16] The personal accountability mentality, which can be perpetuated through medical school education, persists among many. The writer cites a large study conducted in 1984 that found that physicians and physicians in training then believed that they were answerable only to themselves.[17] Many experts comment that health care professionals often view errors as a failure of character.

The Blame-and-Train Approach
As mentioned earlier, many people in contemporary society expect physicians' performance following initial training to be flawless. This feeds the belief that flawed human performance is the root cause of errors. Efforts to retrain personnel following the occurrence of errors or sentinel events focus on eliminating human error. Such efforts also often substitute for a substantive effort to identify, study, and eradicate systems problems. Sometimes called

blame-and-train efforts, they begin with the concept that human error is the source of the problem and that this error is the result of the inattentiveness or insufficiency of practitioners.[18] In his now-classic article "Error in Medicine," Lucian Leape describes role models in medical education—clinical specialists who are authorities—that reinforce the concept of clinician infallibility. According to Leape, the perfectibility model of error prevention is as follows: "If physicians and nurses could be properly trained and motivated, then they would make no mistakes."[19] Using this model, if a nurse made a medication error, she would be punished and retrained. "Although it might be noted that the nurse was distracted because of an unusually large case load, it is unlikely that serious attention would be given to evaluating overall work assignments or to determining if large case loads have contributed to other kinds of errors," writes Leape.[19]

Systems-Oriented Approaches

There *are* effective educational and training approaches that emphasize systems rather than humans as causative factors for errors and the critical preventive role performed by humans. One is the simulated training method used in anesthesiology, described previously. Yet even these approaches are not bulletproof. How can one simulate events that have never happened but could? Or, as error pioneer James Reason asks, how can one simulate events that have not been foreseen?[20]

Reason developed four error management principles that can be applied to many training situations. Those with appropriate controls to ensure patient safety—such as those in simulated environments— are particularly suited to his approach:

- Training should teach and support an active exploratory approach. Trainees should be encouraged to develop their own mental models of the system.
- Error training should form an integral part of the overall training process. Trainees should have the

opportunity to both make errors and recover from them.

- The heuristics of errors should be changed from "mistakes are undesirable" to "it is good to make mistakes; they help learning."
- Error training should be introduced at the appropriate point, midway through a training program. Early in the learning process, trainees are struggling with every step and are unlikely to benefit from error feedback. Later, they are better equipped to learn from such feedback.[20]

Medical school curricula have been changing dramatically during recent years. New curricula are responding to past criticism about a continuing emphasis on memorizing facts, a failure to address the dramatic demands placed on practicing physicians, a continued emphasis on autonomy and the success of the individual (rather than on a team approach), and the absence of curriculum designed to teach students about health care failures. New curricula focus on training physicians for group practice, interdisciplinary team care, and proactive system failure prevention. Two medical educators describe a groundbreaking effort to teach medical students and residents about error in health care.[21] The Michigan State University Kalamazoo Center for Medical Studies developed a curriculum designed to change the blame-and-train mind-set in medical education. "Many of the students/residents commented that this was the first time they understood why they might be involved in quality improvement efforts at the hospital or clinic…. Almost all of the students breathe a sigh of relief when they see the theory behind the mistakes they make, how some of the errors are facilitated by poor design, and the potential for properly designed information systems to help them."[21] Other developments in medical education include small team learning, case-based teaching, earlier introduction to direct contact with patients, and information technology courses.[22]

Needed Curriculum Changes

In the view of many experts, medical education

needs to embrace "system failure education." The second IOM report, *Crossing the Quality Chasm: A New Health System for the 21st Century,* also recommends expanding medical school curriculum to include

- teaching students how to manage knowledge and use effective tools that can support clinical decision making;
- offering more opportunities for multidisciplinary team training in order to reflect the multidisciplinary approach to contemporary medicine; and
- providing clinicians in training with new skills in communication in order to train patients in techniques of good self-management.[15]

Two experts add to this list the study of evidence-based practice and strategies for managing uncertainty.[23] Leape suggests that educational and training efforts should address training for safety as well.[24] According to Leape, physicians and other health care professionals need to be trained how *not to do* things rather than only how *to do* things. Two other experts suggest that conducting root cause analyses on near-miss adverse events can be used as an information source in bringing needed changes to graduate medical education programs.[25]

Continuing Education

The importance of lifelong professional education should permeate undergraduate and graduate medical education. Continuing medical education (CME) for practicing physicians traditionally has focused on professional conferences and the dissemination of medical literature. Morbidity and mortality (M&M) conferences, occurring in hospital settings, aim to teach physicians those principles that might result in the prevention of complications and errors. Their purpose should be an educational one rather than one of finding or ascribing blame. Some indicate that M&M conferences offer the ideal teaching environment that enables physicians and physicians in training an opportunity to intelligently discuss medical and surgical judgment and technique and

patient management issues.[26] Participants should be reassured that adverse outcomes are inevitable and can and should be used in a positive way.[27]

The latest generation of physicians graduating from medical schools is Web-literate. This enhances physicians' ability to stay current with advances as reported in medical literature. Technological tools, such as personal digital assistants (PDAs) and accompanying software enable physicians to easily access such material as practice guidelines and up-to-date drug information. Many graduating physicians work in multidisciplinary practices that emphasize learning from team members.

Risk Management Education

Insurance companies have been proactive in sponsoring loss prevention/risk management activities, including seminars and formal education programs, research studies identifying areas of loss, and site evaluations and office audits aimed at identifying poor clinical and business practices in physicians' offices that can lead to claims experience. Risk management education for physicians and other health care professionals presumes that there are controllable events in medical practice that render a health care professional more or less vulnerable to malpractice claims and that educational efforts focused on such events and on changing practitioner behavior can reduce injury and subsequent claims. "Much of what physicians and other health care providers 'know' about malpractice claims they obtain from water-cooler gossip, poorly prepared media reports, or aggregated data analyses that focus on historical trends rather than on what happened in a particularly incident," suggests one writer.[28] These sources rarely help clinicians learn from others' experiences.

The Harvard Risk Management Foundation (RMF) has championed a program involving the review of closed claim abstracts during grand rounds. "Presenting closed claim abstracts in programs for physicians allows the participants to recognize the important loss prevention points for themselves, without the need for a lecture on 'do's' and 'don'ts.' This format helps disperse the negative emotion that sometimes accompanies discussions of 'what went wrong,'" notes one author.[28] The RMF offers physicians a wide range of online CME courses, such as "The Risks of Poor Communications," "Liability in Medication," and "Documentation Makes the Difference."[29]

Safety-Related Training and Learning

Stephen Small indicates that a compelling case should be made to develop and test safety-related training and to evaluate its impact.[22] Because physicians now function as patient care, information, and team leaders, they must become aware of their role in the system, "learn to manipulate resources for patients' benefit, and develop metacognitive skills— or thinking about thinking—to keep the care path safely on track," writes Small. His thesis is that because safety in complex work is a systems issue, safety training must be advanced as "a component of a systems-level intervention and not simply a provider deficiency." Small concludes that "safety should ultimately be interesting and exciting to practitioners if framed as a component of expert practice, something to which all aspire."[22] Respected clinicians and administrators who will act as role models are vital, notes Small. Sidebar 1-1, page 25, presents a synopsis of his eight suggested principles for developing education and training to improve patient safety.

At the second Annenberg Conference in 1998, researcher-scientist Richard Cook provided a concise summary of the ways in which people and organizations are learning to learn about safety, when he noted the following:

- Learning about safety is not continuous but occurs at intervals.
- Learning requires dissonance between belief and experiences.
- Not everyone learns at the same time.
- Learning is not always sequential.
- Learning does not necessarily produce

appreciation for the consequences of what has been learned.
- Learning about safety is not permanent—it can be forgotten.
- Learning about safety requires close contact with failure and also the distance needed for reflection.
- Learning recapitulates the sequence of research that composes the new outlook on medical errors.
- Learning inherently involves exploring the "second stories" that lie behind accidents and failure.
- Learning about safety exposes organizational stress.
- Learning about safety begins with learning that people make safety.[30]

Education/training and continued professional development related to strategies to reduce and prevent medical failures will help ensure that physicians maintain a leadership role in the improvement of patient safety. The Joint Commission supports the inclusion of patient safety and failure prevention in medical school curricula as an important issue and will be working with educational leaders to help achieve this goal. JCAHO's *Sentinel Event Alerts* (see Sidebar I-3, page 10) aim to provide physicians and all other members of the health care team with ongoing educational information to enhance patient safety. Physicians are advised to use the *Alerts* as a key ongoing information resource.

Proactive Approach 2: Clinical Practice Guidelines

The development and application of clinical practice guidelines by physicians and other health care professionals working in multidisciplinary teams has gained considerable momentum during the past decade as a strategy to help prevent medical failures and thereby enhance patient safety.

A *clinical practice guideline* is a document that describes the processes used to evaluate and treat a patient with a specific diagnosis, condition, or symptom. Found in the literature under many different names, including practice parameters, practice guidelines, patient care protocols, standards

Sidebar 1-1. Suggestions for Developing Education and Training to Improve Patient Safety

1. *Knowledge is power:* Small things do make a difference in complex systems. Safety training need not be prescriptive, but creative. Safety must be fostered by leadership and design but also manifest as a bottom-up provider-take-action phenomenon.

2. *Design systematic safety education and training:* Both are necessary, and not interchangeable. Safety training must use experiential learning techniques and deliberate practice with feedback.

3. *Build on cutting-edge quality improvement and change management know-how:* One cannot assume that individuals arrive ready made with teamwork skills or skills for managing complexity. Improving safety in health care represents a major change in the status quo.

4. *Small-wins approach:* Look for opportunities to begin small, effective projects with a high chance of measurable success and future leverage in the organization.

5. *Emphasize teamwork:* The team is a key unit of analysis for thinking about point-of-care mid-course corrections in complex organizations. Even highly trained experts can benefit from team training if their work is a team task.

6. *Simulate well and often:* Simulation programs hold significant promise as powerful means to deliver both understanding of complexity and metacognitive skills to cope with it.

7. *Horizontal and vertical integration across the organization:* Small interdisciplinary groups (horizontal) and top-to-bottom learning (across the authority gradient) will help break down barriers to understanding microprocesses and build common decision premises, trust, flexibility, and a strong safety culture.

8. *Integrate into ongoing efforts:* Rather than designing and trying to insert a block of safety practice into an already full schedule, imagine ways to knit advanced safety conversations into the fabric of the organization using ongoing M&M conferences, ethics curricula, rounds, CME, and other venues.

Source: Adapted from Small SD: Principles for developing education and training to improve patient safety. *Forum* 21:10–12, Summer 2001. Used with permission. M&M, morbidity and mortality; CME, continuing medical education.

of practice, clinical pathways, and care maps, clinical practice guidelines are designed to reduce variation in the care provided by practitioners, thereby reducing the likelihood of medical failures. Clinical practice guidelines generally differ from standardized protocols in that the guidelines span the entire range of a process from start to finish. For example, a clinical practice guideline on pain covers pain assessment through pain treatment and monitoring.

Some experts distinguish between clinical practice guidelines and clinical pathways.[31] They note that *clinical practice guidelines* define the right *thing* to do, are focused on quality, are research based, and are most effectively formulated at the national level. By contrast, *clinical pathways* define the right *way* to do the right thing, are focused on efficiency, are process based, and are most effectively formulated at the organization level.

Clinical practice guidelines aim at standardization of practice. When well conceived, they can improve care quality and communication among care providers. Guideline use requires all care team members to consider and understand the overall clinical process and the serial and parallel events that must be accomplished to complete a task or procedure.

JCAHO Requirements

The Joint Commission has developed for hospital leaders standards that consider the use of clinical practice guidelines. These vary to some degree among different categories of providers. They do not require leaders to use clinical practice guidelines; rather, they provide a framework for developing and using criteria when considering and reviewing available guidelines for the services and care provided in the organization. When an organization does put guidelines into use, it should ensure the involvement of all appropriate health professionals in guideline development, review, and approval. Leaders provide physicians and other health care professionals with a process for explaining variations from the clinical practice guidelines. The anticipation and management of variation that occurs in implementing the guideline help to maintain practitioner support and improve the guideline. This aims to address the concern expressed by physicians and other professionals that guidelines force them to practice "cookbook medicine." Guidelines must be flexible enough so that physicians can work outside the defined process when required by specific patient needs, without compromising patient safety.[32]

To increase the success of guideline implementation, JCAHO standards recommend review and any necessary modification by the physicians and other health care professionals who will be using them. In short, users must believe in them. Quality research shows that guidelines that represent the most effective way to treat patients help build the necessary trust.[32]

Joint Commission standards require use of clinical practice guidelines in accredited ambulatory care and network organizations. They provide a framework for developing and using criteria when considering and reviewing available guidelines for the services and care provided in the organization. Appropriate leaders, practitioners, and health care professionals *must* review and approve clinical practice guidelines selected for implementation.

Guideline Sources

Guidelines have proliferated during recent years. To help organize practice guidelines and to identify those with an adequate evidence base, the National Guideline Clearinghouse (NGC), a joint effort of the AHRQ, the AMA, and the American Association of Health Plans, provides online access to evidence-based clinical practice guidelines. Founded in 1999, the NGC already contains approximately 1,000 guidelines. Physicians and other health care professionals can access guidelines by disease, mental disorder, or treatment/intervention category at the NGC's Web site, www.clearinghouse.gov.

Guidelines and Evidence-Based Medicine

As noted in the second IOM report, *Crossing the Quality Chasm: A New Health System for the 21st Century,* "Guidelines vary greatly in the degree to which they are derived from and consistent with the evidence base."[15] One of the IOM's key recommendations is the use of consistent evidence-based decision making by physicians and other clinicians. Excerpts of key passages describing this recommendation, or "rule," follow:

> Patients should receive care based on the best available scientific knowledge. Care should not vary illogically from clinician to clinician or from place to place. . . . In today's health system, it is widely believed that the best care for individuals is based on the training and experience of professionals. The new rule, on the other hand, could be stated: *The best care results from the conscientious, explicit, and judicious use of current best evidence and knowledge of patient values by well-trained, experienced clinicians.*

The new rule calls for standardization around best practices as appropriate for a given patient or the subpopulation to which a patient belongs. Such evidence-based decision making can free clinicians to make choices that science cannot guide—decisions based on relationship; observation; and the other senses, including touch…. The commitment to standardizing excellence—using the best available information—does not begin with a slavish adherence to simplistic practice guidelines. With today's information systems, protocols can incorporate variations based on the individual patient's condition.[15]

The IOM asked the AHRQ to determine and disseminate to clinicians a list of best practices that enhance patient safety. That effort resulted in a 2001 report by Kaveh Shojania and colleagues from the University of California.[33] This report is currently generating considerable controversy around the issues of those safety practice improvements that did and did not make the list and the criteria that should be used to determine best practices for improving patient safety. "[R]igorous proof of efficacy according to the rules of the evidence report is neither necessary nor, in many cases, sufficient for recommending widespread use of a safety practice. In addition, as the report points out, it is not always possible to obtain such evidence," comment Lucian Leape, Donald Berwick, and David Bates.[4] Proof of efficacy in the report by Shojania et al required at least one evidence-based study backing it up, and that study needed to include a concurrent or historical control group.

Leape and his colleagues point out that successful safety initiatives in the fields of aviation and anesthesia were achieved by implementing numerous small improvements that in the aggregate made a difference but that were never proven to be effective change by change, and the smaller changes were not subjected to controlled experiments.[4] Health care leaders will need to determine which practices should be recommended to all clinicians.

Guidelines and the Legal Standard of Care

Do clinical practice guidelines constitute the legal standard of care? If so, and with the proliferation of guidelines, how does a physician know which guidelines to follow? Guidelines are hearsay but, under certain circumstances and depending on applicable state law, may be admissible or used in connection with cross-examination of an expert.[34] There are strong arguments to support the view that guidelines should not establish the legal standard of care. Compliance with practice guidelines will not in the vast majority of states, as a matter of law, conclusively defeat a negligence claim, but it may work to the clinician's advantage—if the guidelines are widely recognized as authoritative. "Conversely, a defendant who has departed from authoritative guidelines may have to explain why in court," notes one author.[34] Of course, as a guideline becomes more and more accepted and used with increasing frequency, it may play a greater role in malpractice cases.

It is clear that patient safety can be improved through standardization of care practices. Physicians must take the lead in developing care protocols or guidelines that are practical, evidence based when possible, and user friendly. Keeping guidelines current represents a significant challenge. Physician champions will be needed to ensure thorough implementation and revision of clinical practice guidelines organizationwide in all types of health care organizations.

Proactive Approach 3: Technological Solutions

A revolution in technology, and particularly information technology, is occurring in the health care industry. According to one physician, "This revolution is responding to the basic problem that medical knowledge, skills, drugs, and devices have advanced faster than our ability to deliver them to patients safely, effectively, and efficiently."[35] Health care organizations also struggle with the issue of the cost of new technology.

Computerized Order Entry

When designed and used properly, technology can aid a practitioner's quest for improved patient safety. Online order entry can reduce system failures and is in use broadly in such areas as intravenous therapy ordering, laboratory testing, and procedure ordering. Technological solutions that reduce the likelihood of medical failures have been particularly impressive in the realm of medication use processes. Computerized physician order entry (CPOE), or "electronic prescribing," is one such solution of particular interest to physicians. CPOE, which has perhaps had the largest impact of any automated intervention, is capable of eliminating many problems associated with prescribing. With electronic prescribing, physicians, while in the office or examination room, use a computer or handheld electronic device to generate a prescription and electronically transfer the order to the pharmacy.

Electronic prescribing can significantly reduce handwriting and transcription errors. It can also ensure that dosage, form, and frequency are appropriate and perform a check for potential drug–drug interactions. Allergy checking is also facilitated, as is checking of key patient information related to proposed medications. "Vital patient and drug-specific information, such as overdose warnings, drug interactions, and allergy alerts, can be presented electronically to the prescriber at the moment of order entry so that potential adverse drug events that would otherwise go unrecognized can easily be avoided," writes Michael Cohen, president of the Institute for Safe Medication Practices (ISMP).[36]

Two studies on the impact of electronic prescribing in hospital units found that CPOE decreased the rate of nonintercepted serious medication errors by 50% to 81%.[37,38] The studies conclude that such systems should be more widely used. The Leapfrog Group, a coalition of more than 100 of the nation's largest public and private health care purchasers and organizations, and the National Patient Safety Partnership, a coalition of private and public health care agencies, also recommend the use of computerized order entry. The Leapfrog Group, in fact, established implementation of a CPOE system as one of the three initial methods hospitals should use to improve patient safety.[39] The Leapfrog Group will assess hospitals' compliance with this standard and use the information for future contracting purposes. Online prescribing is not, however, the panacea for medication errors at the prescribing stage. Errors *can* occur even with online prescribing—for example, when an online prescribing system is not properly integrated with the pharmacy's medication control system.

Clinical Information and Decision Support Systems

Web-based clinical information systems are being developed and implemented at numerous hospitals and hospital systems.[35] Computerized decision support systems (CDSSs) have also been shown to reduce the frequency of adverse drug events.[40] CDSSs are defined as "software that integrates information on the characteristics of individual patients with a computerized knowledge base for the purpose of generating patient-specific assessments or recommendations designed to aid clinicians and/or patients in making clinical decisions."[15] CDSSs can be used to help physicians and other clinicians with preventive and monitoring tasks, prescribing of drugs, and diagnosis and management.[15] Use of CDSSs in acute care settings remains limited, but the IOM believes that greater public investment in research and development in such systems is warranted.[15] Chapter 4 further describes CPOE and other strategies to reduce medication-related failures.

Automation and Failures

Computerization and automation are not bulletproof. Automation can effectively prevent failures by pausing the process when an error is detected. This gives humans the required time to intervene and address the problem.[41] However, automation and the improper use of automated devices, alarms, or other equipment can increase practitioner errors. Equipment might not work in the way the user expects, or the practitioner may use the technology improperly because of insufficient training and opportunity to practice prior to use.[42] Alarms for patient monitoring might be turned off because they have high rates of false alarms, or practitioners might "burn out" because of alarm noises. "One wonders whether the design of alarms is driven by what is technically possible and by legal concerns, as opposed to by the requirements for providing relevant and timely information to human operators," note two writers.[43]

Alarms and other medical equipment or devices also might malfunction because of user or technical problems. Recognizing the critical role played by proactive alarm maintenance and testing, one of JCAHO's National Patient Safety Goals for 2003 is to "improve the effectiveness of clinical alarm systems" by implementing regular preventive maintenance and testing and by assuring that alarms are activated with appropriate settings and are sufficiently audible with respect to distances and competing noise within the unit.[44] Problems with alarm systems were cited as a root cause of sentinel events in 8% of the sentinel events reviewed by JCAHO.[45]

Competence and Technology Usage

To ensure patient safety, physicians must be competent in the use of the required technology. Health care organizations verify such competence through the credentialing and privileging process.* The importance of credentialing and privileging cannot be overstated. Two of the most crucial tasks performed in health care facilities, they are designed to help ensure the organization and its patients that the patients will receive safe, quality care. As a consequence of the rapid explosion of medical knowledge, the resulting era of specialized medicine,

---

* *Credentialing* is the process of obtaining, verifying, and assessing the qualifications of a health care practitioner to provide patient care services in or for a health care organization. *Privileging* is the process whereby a specific scope and content of patient care services (that is, clinical privileges) are authorized for a health care practitioner by a health care organization based on evaluation of the individual's credentials and performance.

and the litigious nature of modern society, health care organizations must ensure that the practitioners providing care within their walls are both qualified and competent. Patient health care outcomes are tied directly to these factors.

With the increase in available technology, diagnostic and therapeutic options are changing rapidly. These new developments often render some clinical approaches outdated while they make new ones available. The health care organization's medical staff must periodically review the entire range of privileges authorized and practiced within the facility to ensure that the determination actually reflects the practice within the organization and that it is appropriate to the needs of the community it serves. The use of new, specialized technology is a critical area that requires regular review.

Proactive Approach 4: Collaboration and Communication

Traditionally, teamwork or collaboration among health care professionals has not been stressed in the health care environment. Physicians, placing a high degree of value on autonomy, are trained to think as individuals rather than as team members. The second IOM report notes, "In the current system, care is taken to protect professional prerogatives and separate roles. The current system shows too little cooperation and teamwork…. That approach makes defined roles preeminent rather than meeting patients' needs."[15]

This worldview is changing and needs to continue to do so dramatically. As part of a comprehensive error reduction and prevention strategy, health care organizations are recognizing the importance of groups functioning as teams and are creating interdisciplinary teams or task forces charged with improving organizational performance to reduce medical failures. Teamwork is important not only in complex and dynamic environments such as ORs and EDs, but also throughout patient care functions and processes. Teamwork operates on the assumption that collective knowledge, skill, and wisdom will be greater than what one individual could bring to the table.[46] Physicians must assume a leadership role in such multidisciplinary teams to protect patients from harm.

The Dangers of a Hierarchical Culture

Coordination of care among health care professionals through an interdisciplinary care-management process and coordinated communication are vital to safety. Yet all too often, organization leaders need to give interdisciplinary collaboration a higher priority. Fiefdoms and hierarchical "pecking orders" interfere with properly coordinated care focused on meeting individuals' needs. "It is clear that the structure of authority in teams and groups is critically important in reducing error. If a team has a very strong hierarchy, then it will be difficult for juniors to question decisions made by those at a higher level of authority even when the latter make errors. Furthermore, there will be a tendency for those low in the hierarchy to be afraid to show initiative," notes Neville Moray.[46] A hierarchical culture makes nurses and all other health care professionals reluctant to raise concerns or question physicians about issues that could result in patient injury.

The Role of Staffing Shortages

Reduced staffing experienced in most health care organizations today heightens the critical need for a multidisciplinary approach to error reduction. Authors write, "Reduced staffing has forced us to acknowledge professional interdependence and the need for collaboration among physicians, pharmacists, nurses, and patients."[47] The increasing prevalence of patients with chronic conditions who need a mix of services over time and across settings also heightens the need for a multidisciplinary approach to medical care.[15]

In August 2002 the Joint Commission released a white paper titled "Health Care at the Crossroads: Strategies for Addressing the Evolving Nursing Crisis."[48] This paper is a product of a JCAHO Public

Policy Initiative that seeks to address broad issues that have the potential to seriously undermine the provision of safe, high-quality health care. The white paper is a call to action for those who influence, develop, or carry out policies that will lead the way to resolution of the issue. Nurse shortage solutions identified by JCAHO target three areas: creating a culture of retention, bolstering nursing education, and establishing financial incentives for investing in nursing. Although the report focuses on the nursing shortages, it acknowledges other compelling shortages of health care personnel, including pharmacists, radiological technologists, laboratory technologists, billing/coders, and respiratory therapists. Staffing shortages are acute not only in hospitals but also throughout health care settings. They affect all caregivers in all health care settings.

Changing the Culture

Health care leaders must ensure an environment and culture conducive to communication and collaboration, and physicians must be a part of that leadership effort. In its February 2000 report to the president, the QuIC Task Force wrote:

> Because of the nature of medical errors, an effective response requires an integration of efforts across traditional occupational and scientific boundaries. The nature of the patient safety challenge requires synergy among scientific and technical disciplines, from human factors psychology to product design and delivery. This collaboration is needed at all stages of the effort to reduce errors and enhance patient safety—from research on its causes and remedies to implementation and partnership in its reduction and elimination.[49]

Physicians' collaboration as integral members of multidisciplinary teams is essential to the way care is now provided. Physicians are responsible for participating in organizationwide performance improvement teams to investigate the root causes of medical failures that have occurred and proactively working to identify and implement failure reduction opportunities. Some physicians express concern about the time involved in such endeavors, worried that such efforts take time away from direct patient care. Yet because care of patients is physicians' first priority, their involvement in these safety-related efforts is critical and must be considered part of the care they provide. Strategies to make the best use of physicians' time, such as the use of voicemail and e-mail to keep physicians informed of team discussions and their attendance only during key decision-making meetings, can be explored.

Communication Improvement

The need for improved and increased communication by and among physicians and other health care professionals warrants special focus. Communication failures were cited in 63% of all sentinel events reviewed by the Joint Commission since 1995, making this the most frequently occurring problem associated with all types of sentinel events. Communication was the first or second root cause cited for operative and postoperative errors and complications, medication errors, wrong-site surgery, delays in treatment, falls, and home care fires. Communication failures must be viewed as having systems roots rather than as being attributable to any specific health care professional, but health care professionals must ensure that they are communicating with their colleagues as true team members.

Physician–Patient Communication

In addition to communication among physicians and other health care professionals, communication among physicians and patients and their families is essential to medical care and to improved patient safety. Citing earlier studies,[50,51] two experts write:

> Evidence has shown that communication skills can be taught and can have a positive effect on consultation behaviours such as active listening and empathy, and that outcomes such as patient satisfaction improve as patients become more equal partners in the doctor–patient relationship. Medical student communication skills training, emphasizing the benefits of mutualistic, enabling doctor behaviours, could therefore lead to a

greater valuing of the lay perspective and perhaps less medical emphasis on the exclusivity of professional judgement.[23]

The patient is a partner to the physician in the care process when things are going well *and* when things do not go as well as expected. This means that physicians are required to explain to the patient and/or the patient's family unanticipated care outcomes. Physicians and other clinicians also need to have skills to train patients in self-management techniques for chronic conditions.[15] "Unfortunately, many physicians see themselves only as technicians and fail to see their role as teacher, advocate, and companion. In this regard, physicians need to become better listeners," notes one writer.[52] Although one might argue with this writer's use of the word *many*, it is fair to say that most physicians do struggle with the multiple hats they must wear.

Patients and family members also must be educated about the value of increased communication with care providers. The Joint Commission's Speak Up campaign, described earlier, encourages patients and families to inform caregivers if they have questions or concerns about some aspect of care. Patient safety often depends on high-quality patient/family–provider communication.

Concluding Comments

Clearly, physicians must play a leadership role in proactively improving systems and processes to reduce the likelihood of medical failures that could harm patients in all types of health care organizations. Education, technology, physician-driven clinical practice guidelines, teamwork, and communication represent major improvement opportunities. The following chapters outline specific strategies and practices that support the provision of team-based, efficient, safe, high-quality care to patients in order to reduce operative and postoperative errors and complications; wrong-site, wrong-patient, and wrong-procedure surgery; medication errors; treatment delays; serious injury or death from physical restraints, and suicide.

REFERENCES

1. Starr P: *The Social Transformation of American Medicine.* New York: Basic Books, Inc, 1982, p 22.

2. Joint Commission: Engaging physicians in the performance improvement process. *Jt Comm Persp* 21:8–9, Jul 2001.

3. Ketring SP, White JP: Developing a systemwide approach to patient safety. *Jt Comm J Qual Improv* 28:287–95, Jun 2002.

4. Leape LL, Berwick DM, Bates DW: What practices will most improve safety? Evidence-based medicine meets patient safety. *JAMA* 288:501–7, 24/31 Jul 2002.

5. Cooper JB, et al: Effects of information feedback and pulse oximetry on the incidence of anesthesia complications. *Anesthesiology* 67:686–94, 1987.

6. Forrest J, et al: Multicenter study of general anesthesia. II. Results. *Anesthesiology* 72(2):262–8, 1990.

7. Bogner MS (ed): *Human Error in Medicine.* Hillsdale, NJ: Lawrence Erlbaum Associates, 1994, p 9.

8. Cooper JB, et al: Preventable anesthesia mishaps: A study of human factors. *Anesthesiology* 49(6):399–406, 1978.

9. Gaba D, Maxwell M, DeAnda A: Anesthetic mishaps: Breaking the chain of accident evolution. *Anesthesiology* 66(5):670–6, 1987.

10. Gaba DM: Anaesthesiology as a model for patient safety in health care. *BMJ* 320:785–8, 18 Mar 2000.

11. Spencer FC: Human error in hospitals and industrial accidents: Current concepts. *J Am Coll Surg* 191:410–8, Oct 2000.

12. Tinker JH, et al: Role of monitoring devices in prevention of anesthetic mishaps: A closed claims analysis. *Anesthesiology* 71:541–6, Oct 1989.

13. Cooper JB, Newbower RS, Ritz RJ: An analysis of major errors and equipment failures in anesthesia management—Considerations for prevention and detection. *Anesthesiology* 60(1):34–42, 1984.

14. Gaba DM, DeAnda A: The response of anesthesia trainees to simulated critical incidents. *Anesth Analga* 68(4):444–51, 1989.

15. Institute of Medicine: *Crossing the Quality Chasm: A New Health System for the 21st Century.* Washington, DC: National Academy Press, 2001.

16. Sharpe VA: "No tribunal other than his own conscience": Historical reflections on harm and responsibility in medicine. Presented at Enhancing Patient Safety and Reducing Errors in Health Care (Annenberg II), Rancho Mirage, CA, 8 Nov 1998.

17. Mizrahi T: Managing medical mistakes: Ideology, insularity and accountability among internists in training. *Soc Sci Med* 19(2):135–46, 1984.

18. Cook RI, Woods DD: Operating at the sharp end: The complexity of human error. In Bogner MS (ed): *Human Error in Medicine.* Hillsdale, NJ: Lawrence Erlbaum Associates, 1994, p 301.

19. Leape LL: Error in medicine. *JAMA* 272:1851–57, 21 Dec 1994.

20. Reason J: *Human Error.* Cambridge: Cambridge University Press, 1990, pp 245–6.

21. Gosbee J, Stahlhut R: Teaching medical students and residents about error in health care. Presented at Enhancing Patient Safety and Reducing Errors in Health Care (Annenberg I), Rancho Mirage, CA, Oct 1996.

22. Small SD: Principles for developing education and training to improve patient safety. *Forum* 21:10–2, summer 2001.

23. Lester H, Tritter JQ: Medical error: A discussion of the medical construction of error and suggestions for reforms of medical education to decrease error. *Medical Education* 35:855–61, Sep 2001.

24. Leape LL: Errors in health care—Problems and challenges. Presented at Enhancing Patient Safety and Reducing Errors in Health Care (Annenberg I), Rancho Mirage, CA, Oct 1996.

25. Battles JB, Shea CE: A system of analyzing medical errors to improve GME curricula and programs. *Acad Med* 76:125–33, Feb 2001.

26. Murayama KM, et al: A critical evaluation of the morbidity and mortality conference. *Am J Surg* 183:246–50, Mar 2002.

27. Harbison S, Regehr G: Faculty and resident opinions regarding the role of morbidity and mortality conference. *Am J Surg* 177:136–9, Feb 1999.

28. Martin PB: Using closed malpractice claims as teaching tools. *Forum* 18:1, Mar 1998.

29. Risk Management Foundation CME Online. Web site: www.rmf.harvard.edu/edprograms/cme-online/body.html.

30. Cook RI: Two years before the mast: Learning how to learn about patient safety. Presented at Enhancing Patient Safety and Reducing Errors in Health Care (Annenberg II), Rancho Mirage, CA, 8–10 Nov 1998.

31. Miller CF, Dolter KJ: Evidence-based condition management: DoD/VA clinical practice guidelines—Tools to effect best practices. Presented at the 2001 TRICARE Conference, Washington, DC, 24 Jan 2001.

32. Medication safety issue brief 5: Crucial role of therapeutic guidelines. *Hosp Health Netw* 75:65–6, May 2001.

33. Shojania K, et al (eds): *Making Health Care Safer: A Critical Analysis of Patient Safety Practices.* Rockville, MD: Agency for Healthcare Research and Quality, 2001. Web site: www.ahqr.gov.

34. Mello MM: Commentary: The role of clinical practice guidelines in malpractice litigation. *Forum* 20:1, Fall 2000.

35. Ricci R: Use the right stuff the right way. *Modern Healthcare* 32:27, 8 Jul 2002.

36. Cohen MR (ed): *Medication Errors.* Washington, DC: American Pharmaceutical Association, 1999, p 8.19.

37. Bates DW, et al: Effect of computerized physician order entry and a team intervention on prevention of serious medication errors. *JAMA* 280(15):1311–6, 1998.

38. Bates DW, et al: The impact of computerized physician order entry on medication error prevention. *J Am Med Inform Assoc* 6(4):313–21, 1999.

39. Sarudi D: The leapfrog effect. *Hosp Health Netw* 75:32–6, May 2001.

40. Evans RS, et al: A computer-assisted management program for antibiotics and other anti-infective agents. *NEJM* 338:232–8, 1998.

41. Spath PL: Reducing errors through work system improvements. In Spath PL (ed): *Error Reduction in Health Care: A Systems Approach to Improving Patient Safety.* San Francisco: Jossey-Bass, 2000, p 225.

42. VanCott H: Human errors: Their causes and reduction. In Bogner MS (ed): *Human Error in Medicine.* Hillsdale, NJ: Lawrence Erlbaum Associates, 1994, p 58.

43. Xiao Y, Seagull J: Toward a user friendly health care environment: The case of alarms. *Forum* 21:17–8, Summer 2001.

44. Joint Commission: JCAHO approves National Patient Safety Goals for 2003. *Jt Comm Persp* 22:1–3, Sep 2002.

45. Joint Commission: Statistics provide insight into causes of sentinel events. *Jt Comm Persp* 22:3–5, Aug 2002.

46. Moray N: Error reduction as a systems problem. In Bogner MS (ed): *Human Error in Medicine.* Hillsdale, NJ: Lawrence Erlbaum Associates, 1994, p 79.

47. Knox GE, et al: Downsizing, reengineering and patient safety: Numbers, new-ness and resultant risk. *J Health Risk Manag* 19:18–25, Fall 1999.

48. Joint Commission: *Health Care at the Crossroads: Strategies for Addressing the Evolving Nursing Crisis* (white paper). Oakbrook Terrace, IL, Aug 2002.

49. Quality Interagency Coordination Task Force: *Doing what counts for patient safety: Federal actions to reduce medical errors and their impact.* Report to the President, Feb 2000. Web site: www.quic.gov.

50. Usherwood T: Subjective and behavioural evaluation of the teaching of patient interview skills. *Med Educ* 27:41–7, Jan 1993.

51. Coulter A: Partnerships with patients: The pros and cons of shared clinical decision-making. *J Health Serv Res Policy* 2:112–21, Apr 1997.

52. Clark PA: What residents are not learning: Observations in an NICU. *Acad Med* 76:419–24, May 2001.

PROTECTING PATIENTS FROM OPERATIVE AND POSTOPERATIVE ERRORS AND COMPLICATIONS

Nowhere is the advance of contemporary medicine more apparent than in modern-day ORs and surgical suites. Once unimaginable feats, such as the simultaneous transplantation of multiple organs and the permanent correction of vision, occur daily if not routinely in thousands of surgical settings.

As noted earlier, OR environments are complex and dynamic, with constant change and time pressures. Operative procedures require the effort of physicians, nurses, and technicians working smoothly as a team. Issues relevant to prevention of sentinel events start well before the patient arrives in the OR. With the extensive and increasing use of outpatient surgery, health care professionals working in the office, clinic, and extended care facility might be involved in numerous prevention issues.

This chapter addresses system failures and prevention strategies relevant for physicians as leaders of a health care team throughout a surgical patient's care continuum.

Cause for Concern

The past decades have witnessed a dramatic increase in the number and types of operative procedures. As operative volume—now estimated to be greater than 40 million each year—increases, so does the risk of sentinel events. More than ten years ago, the now-classic Harvard Medical Practice Study analyzed all serious adverse events in hospitalized patients.[1] Although that research considered much more than

sentinel events, the data revealed that 48% of the adverse events were related to surgery. Wound infections were the most common surgical adverse events, accounting for 29% of surgical complications and nearly one-seventh of all adverse events identified in the study.

A study following the Harvard study, conducted at the University of Chicago, indicated that about 20% of serious adverse events were related to surgery and that avoidable adverse events occurred in 18% of the admissions.[2] These findings are very similar to those of a California Medical Association study conducted more than a decade earlier.[3] In the Chicago study, half the potential compensable events were found to result from treatment in the OR. Data collected among health care consumers confirm the frequency of adverse events related to surgical or operative procedures. The public opinion poll conducted for the NPSF found that 22% of patients surveyed had experienced mistakes during medical (or surgical) procedures.[4]

Because of the high risks associated with surgery, some loss-prevention specialists estimate that a surgeon's annual probability of being named in a malpractice claim or suit may soon reach 1 in 20.[5] A sampling of surgical adverse events that had payments in excess of $1 million for one malpractice carrier includes the following: infection following hysterectomy; severed popliteal artery by drill; perforation of the eye; and hematoma following surgery, resulting in paralysis.[5] "Litigation aside, the costs of surgical adverse events include further

Table 2-1. Complications of Operative and Other Invasive Procedures

- Insertion of nasogastric/feeding tubes into the trachea or a bronchus;
- Massive fluid overload during genitourinary/gynecological procedures due to the absorption of irrigation fluids;
- Acute respiratory failure and cardiac arrest during open orthopedic operations;
- Perforation of adjacent organs during endoscopic procedures, including nongastrointestinal procedures (for example, lacerations of the liver were among the most frequent complications of thoracic and abdominal endoscopic operations);
- Central venous catheter insertion into an artery;
- Liver lacerations, peritonitis, or respiratory arrest as the result of an imaging-directed percutaneous biopsy or tube placement; and
- Burns from electrocautery used with a flammable prep solution.

Source: Joint Commission: Operative and postoperative complications: Lessons for the future. *Sentinel Event Alert* Issue 12, 4 Feb 2000.

operations, extended lengths of stay, additional outpatient visits, and decreased trust in the health care system. Looking beyond the individuals to the systems that may have set clinicians up to fail is vitally important," says one expert.[5]

Data from the Joint Commission's sentinel event database, including more than 1,600 sentinel events reviewed by the organization from January 1995 through May 2002, indicate that operative and postoperative errors and complications accounted for 12.2% of sentinel events.[6] Only suicide (17.1%) surpassed operative and postoperative errors and complications as a proportion of the total. Suicides

in fact may be reported most often because they are impossible to overlook. As of May 2002, 200 operative or postoperative errors or complications had been reviewed by JCAHO.

A *Sentinel Event Alert* on suicide, published in 2000 by the Joint Commission, revealed that of the operative and postoperative sentinel events in acute care hospitals reviewed by the Joint Commission, 84% resulted in deaths and 16% resulted in serious injury.[7] These data specifically excluded cases directly related to medication errors, the administration of anesthesia, and wrong-site surgery. The complications occurred during the induction of anesthesia (6%), intraoperatively (23%), during postanesthesia recovery (13%), and postoperatively (58%). Only 10% of the cases were considered emergencies. The procedures involved numerous specialties, such as interventional imaging or endoscopy, tube or catheter insertion, open abdominal surgery, orthopedic surgery, head and neck surgery, and thoracic surgery. The most frequent complications are listed in Table 2-1, left.

The Physician's Role

The surgeon is front and center during the operative process, preoperative assessment, and postoperative monitoring. The surgeon creates the care plan, leads the operative team through performance of the required procedure(s), and serves as the patient's and family's key contact throughout the surgery and recuperative process. Describing the best possible surgical environment, Lucian Leape notes, "Watching a good surgeon can be a real delight. There is a minimum of unnecessary motion, things go smoothly, and everyone knows what to do. They have an efficient team. They have standardized the process and simplified it, and they have made it elegant."[8]

One physician describes the environment experienced by many senior surgeons, who perhaps have been working in smaller cities and smaller hospitals. These surgeons have spent much of their professional careers working in the same OR with

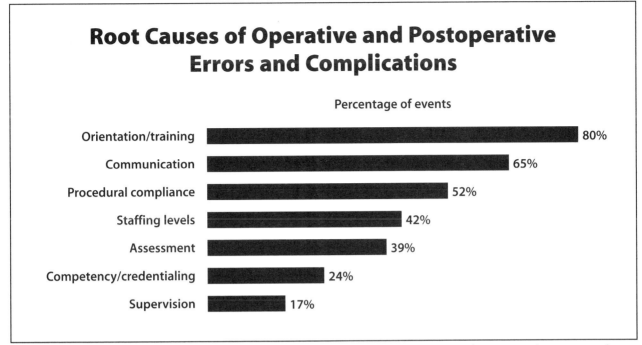

Root Causes of Operative and Postoperative Errors and Complications

Percentage of events

Orientation/training	80%
Communication	65%
Procedural compliance	52%
Staffing levels	42%
Assessment	39%
Competency/credentialing	24%
Supervision	17%

Figure 2-1. This chart illustrates the percentage of causes at the root of operative and postoperative errors and complications-related sentinel events reported to the Joint Commission between January 1995 and May 2002. Source: Joint Commission: Statistics provide insight into causes of sentinel events. *Jt Comm Persp* 22:3–5, Aug 2002.

the same nurses and anesthesiologists.[9] They are familiar with OR protocol and each other's expectations. As the physician notes, however,

> That is rarely the situation in major hospitals today, particularly in the major teaching hospitals. The surgeon who sees the same anesthesiologist or nursing team every day is fortunate. Certainly, if emergency surgery is required "off hours," a group of highly trained strangers is gathered, rather than a highly trained and experienced team. Even though everyone involved may be talented, they are not a team. The absence of strict protocols, not just "doctor preference cards," denies the patient a critical safety factor.[9]

Successful operation and postoperative recovery require a high-quality health care team. Staffing, training and competency, information availability and exchange, equipment and materials, communication, and collaboration each present a system-based challenge that must be met to ensure patient safety.

Common Systems Failures

The causes of sentinel events due to operative and postoperative errors and complications cross disciplinary boundaries and reflect systems failures. Organizations experiencing operative and postoperative sentinel events reviewed by the Joint Commission to date identified the following as root causes:

- Incomplete communication among caregivers;
- Failure to follow established procedures;
- Necessary personnel not being available when needed;
- Incomplete preoperative assessment;
- Deficiencies in credentialing and privileging;
- Inadequate supervision of house staff;
- Inconsistent postoperative monitoring procedures; and
- Failure to question inappropriate orders.[7]

Figure 2-1, above, illustrates the frequency of occurrence of the key root causes. A review of key root causes and the responsibilities of physicians as team leaders and members is critical to the successful development and implementation of effective error prevention strategies to protect the patient from harm.

System Solution 1: Communication and Information Management

Sentinel Event Example: Insufficient Sharing of Information

A patient has a central venous line inserted while waiting in his hospital room prior to going to the OR. The surgical resident orders a chest x-ray to determine the position of the catheter. Before the results of the x-ray are available, the surgical resident has to leave the area to attend to a serious situation in the ED. After the patient is sent to the OR, the unit clerk on the patient's floor receives the radiology report and posts the report in the patient's box. The report indicates the presence of a dangerous pneumothorax.

The information concerning the pneumothorax is not sent to the OR because radiology does not communicate the urgency of the report. The unit clerk does not know what information should be directed to the OR. The staff in the OR does not note that a piece of vital information is missing. The patient suffers a cardiopulmonary arrest during the procedure.

This example demonstrates the critical importance of well-established communication channels and thorough information management processes and procedures that address priority information sent and received. Two-thirds of the organizations reporting to the Joint Commission sentinel events due to operative and postoperative errors and complications identified incomplete communication among caregivers as a root cause. Usually a patient undergoing an operative procedure comes into contact with multiple members of an organization's staff and health care providers in the community. Physicians help create a climate that is conducive to a team approach characterized by open and honest communication about issues and information relevant to patient safety.

Organization leaders must clearly define expected channels of communication. Direct communication among health care providers is obviously the optimal method for preventing mishaps. But because it is not always possible, the need for other accurate and precise methods of communication, such as documentation, must be considered and developed. Many organizations have found that the use of multidisciplinary progress notes improves communication among health care providers and makes care plans more useful. Having all the progress notes from each practitioner in the same area of the record makes it is easier to identify what is incomplete or missing. Multidisciplinary progress notes also increase the relevance and use of the care plans.

Often, different departments or divisions develop forms to document their activities. However, department outsiders may not be able to interpret the comments, abbreviations, or terminology used in the form. Efforts to standardize terminology, definitions, vocabulary, nomenclature, abbreviations, and symbols should be undertaken by an interdisciplinary team. Failure to do so invites error. A table that provides abbreviations, symbols, and their meanings could be kept with patients' clinical records for ease of reference.

Documentation aids communication. For example, often a nurse must communicate to a physician information from a radiology report that confirms the correct placement of a catheter. Failure to communicate the results of a confirmation procedure has led to misplacement of tubes and catheters. The confirmation report also may be sent to a long term care facility if the patient is transferred shortly after the catheter placement. Communication through this document enhances care continuity throughout the continuum of care. Requiring an operative progress note to be entered in the medical record immediately after surgery reduces the likelihood of postoperative complications. Properly documented care plans help to ensure optimal patient care and communication among all caregivers.

Maintain open, consistent, and direct communication with preoperative and surgical staff. Direct communication among physicians and other health care providers is essential to the prevention of sentinel events due to operative and postoperative errors and complications. Surgeons and anesthesiologists must allow and even encourage members of the operative team to question orders, without becoming defensive. They can encourage second opinions. Nurses and other members of the surgical team must feel comfortable enough about established communication channels to promptly and freely question physician orders that they feel may be inappropriate or unclear. A hierarchical approach to medical care must be replaced by a teamwork approach. To facilitate clear communication, physicians should ask staff to write down instructions and read back the care instructions for confirmation by the physician. Phone calls and pages from staff most often require physician response. "Value all communication, regardless of position and rank," advises one expert.[5]

 Maintain open, consistent, and direct communication with patient and family. Physicians communicate with the patient and family about the diagnosis, intended treatment, and possible care outcomes through the informed consent process. To ensure realistic and accurate patient expectations, physicians ask the patient and/or family members to repeat their understanding of operative procedures, follow-up activities, and expected care outcomes. Physicians can ask confirmatory questions. Communication trouble spots identified by a risk management expert, include not listening or not paying attention to the patient's preferences; not evaluating patients promptly; not returning phone calls; inadequate discussion of alternatives to surgery and risks of complications; and failure to prepare patients for the realities of surgery, that is, closing the "expectation gap."[5] "Improving the patient's decision making process is paramount," the expert notes. Many surgery malpractice cases result from "inadequate

explanations of risks and repeated failures to communicate with the patient and family."[5] The patient's and family's concerns should be addressed as thoroughly as possible.

Physicians might wish to seek guidance about how to inform the patient and family member of unfavorable care outcomes following treatment. See information on pages 13 and 14 related to Joint Commission requirements for informing patients and family members of unanticipated outcomes of care and one organization's procedure for medical accident disclosure (Sidebar I-4).

 Obtain and integrate into decision making all key information relevant to the patient's safe care. Physicians must be equipped with all appropriate information relevant to the case at hand. X-rays, medical records, consultative reports, and other diagnostic studies provide the data needed for timely and high-quality decision making and safe, effective care. "Surgery cases (with adverse outcomes) related to clinical judgment arose from many factors that left clinicians lacking information they needed at key decision points," notes an expert.[5] Among other examples of factors, this expert cites incomplete or inaccurate history taking, overreliance on the referring physician's diagnosis without independent assessment, failure to obtain consultation, poor office systems for tracking test results, and misinterpretation of diagnostic studies.

 Share with the care team all information relevant to the patient's safe care. Incomplete information sharing among surgical team members increases the likelihood of adverse outcomes. For example, a surgeon needs to brief OR team members about the operative plan and any expected or possible variations.

 Use documentation as a communication tool. Physicians are often reminded of the importance of good documentation. Thorough documentation can reduce the likelihood of sentinel events—for example, by informing other team members that a medication that requires close monitoring has been ordered for the patient. Certainly, inadequate or missing documentation reflects unfavorably on the provider's overall competence and ability to provide safe patient care. As feasible, physicians can teach other staff how to read physicians' reports. For example, following physician-led training related to interpreting the anesthesia record in a facility, nurses were able to identify specific events during the administration of anesthesia, review vital signs, identify medications and fluids used, and understand and help implement plans for the recovery period.

With all documentation, legible handwriting is essential. Joint Commission standards require author authentication of entries to history and physical examinations, operative procedures, consultations, and discharge summaries. Indications of authentication can include written signatures or initials, rubber stamps, or computer signatures.

 Use clinical practice guidelines to enhance communication. When available and appropriate, clinical practice guidelines provide a means to improve care quality and communication and enhance utilization of health care services. Guideline use requires all care team members to consider and understand the overall clinical process and the serial and parallel events that must be accomplished to complete a task or procedure. Practice guidelines offer an excellent opportunity to guarantee that the needed communication issues are addressed. (See also previous discussion in Chapter 1.)

System Solution 2: Competence and Staffing

Sentinel Event Example: Inadequate Training

An orthopedic surgeon, covering one evening for his partner, arrives in an ED to care for a patient with a dislocated shoulder. The surgeon rarely performs elective procedures at this facility but does so and is privileged to do so in neighboring facilities. He indicates that he intends to use conscious sedation, which he has used before, while setting the patient's shoulder. The surgeon was unaware that the hospital recently instituted a program for physician training, testing, and privileging in conscious sedation and that new data related to assessing risk prior to instituting conscious sedation were provided at that program. The patient's obesity and problems with sleep apnea are clear indicators that the patient is at increased risk for an adverse outcome. However, the surgeon is not aware of these risk factors. He commences the procedure. The patient experiences a respiratory arrest. A review of the surgeon's credentials and privileges reveals that he did not attend the hospital's training program and was not privileged at the facility for conscious sedation.

Organizations experiencing sentinel events related to operative and postoperative procedures most frequently cite staff orientation and training and clinical competence and credentialing as root causes. Delineation of clinical privileges by medical staff leaders outlines the techniques and procedures each practitioner is privileged to perform in that facility. Although the surgeon in the example above might have been privileged to perform conscious sedation in other hospitals, his privileges did not extend to the facility in this example.

Credentialing, privileging, training, competence, and staff adequacy are leadership issues. An adequate number of staff members with the experience and training necessary must be available to meet patient care needs. This Joint Commission requirement is addressed in the "Management of Human Resources" function of all accreditation programs, stating, "The organization provides an adequate number of staff members whose qualifications are consistent with job responsibilities." The special training required for various operations or procedures makes staffing a challenge in most hospitals and ambulatory care settings.

Many organizations maintain generic competencies lists and job descriptions for categories of employees. These do not meet the requirements outlined in Joint Commission "Management of Human Resources" standards. Job descriptions and competence requirements must accurately reflect the job being performed. Accurate and specific requirements serve as guidelines for orientation, training, and competence assessment. As outlined in the "Medical Staff," "Improving Organization Performance," and "Management of Human Resources" chapters of all accreditation manuals, medical staff and other leaders must continuously assess competence through the recredentialing and reprivileging processes or performance evaluation process, collect and analyze data on competence patterns, and determine continuing professional education needs. The data collection must be based on a meaningful evaluation process that assesses each staff member's ability to meet performance expectations outlined in the person's job description or privilege delineation. Generic evaluation forms can assess only the basics. Specific tasks, especially those involving procedures and equipment, must be evaluated. Assessment of age-specific competence should include actual observation of specific tasks related to the patients involved.

Obtain high-quality training.

Anesthesiologists' training includes use of simulation that allows individuals in training to learn to respond to unexpected emergency scenarios. Surgical training lacks full-scale simulators that model the entire range of anatomies and possible adverse incidents. For example, "training in cardiac surgery comprises observation and assistance with cases, combined with lecturing and seminars from senior surgeons," describes one team of authors.[10] Because there are no full-scale simulators of the heart, "the junior surgeon may not be given the opportunity to learn about infrequently occurring and unusual coronary arterial patterns that make the surgical procedure more complicated."[10] In new areas of surgical practice or areas that have changed in major ways, surgeons with less experience can work in tandem with someone on staff who has extensive experience in this methodology and has demonstrated competency in the procedure to be performed.

Ensure appropriate credentials and privileges for procedures performed.

A physician or other practitioner should know when arriving on a unit requesting to perform an invasive procedure whether he or she is privileged to perform that procedure in that facility. Health care organizations should have a mechanism for identifying privileges held by each practitioner. Although this places the staff in an often uncomfortable position, timely checking can help prevent sentinel events. During the day, a nurse manager can usually check with the medical staff office. However, in the evening, that might not be possible, so other mechanisms must be provided.

Revise the credentialing, privileging, and competence evaluation process.

Medical staff leaders should ensure a thorough competence evaluation process for all LIPs practicing under the organization's aegis. If the process is not thorough, it should be revised. The assessment process focuses initially on verification of current competence and the ability to perform requested privileges and/or assume an appointment to the medical staff. After the individual has been appointed and/or granted privileges, the focus shifts to ongoing monitoring of competence through a variety of mechanisms, such as peer review, reprivileging, and recredentialing. Also, an analysis should be conducted of the volume of procedures performed. "One size fits all" credentialing is not permitted by the Joint Commission.

The importance of credentialing and privileging cannot be overstated. As two of the most crucial tasks performed in health care facilities, they are designed to help assure the organization's staff and its patients that the patients will receive quality care. With the dramatic growth of medical knowledge, the resulting era of specialized medicine, and the litigious nature of modern society, health care organizations must ensure that the practitioners providing care within their walls are both qualified and competent. Patient health care outcomes are tied directly to these factors. Sidebar 2-1, page 43 provides more information on credentialing and privileging.

 Inform leaders of unsafe staffing situations. Physicians must communicate their concern about unsafe staffing situations, due either to improperly trained operative team members or to an inadequate number or mix of team members. If physicians believe that staffing issues could compromise patient safety, they should not proceed with the surgery. The lack of availability of necessary trained personnel has been cited as a root cause of many operative and postoperative errors and complications. Surgical assistants not properly trained for cardiac surgery, for example, can cause "tension errors" when they do not hold the organ at the correct level of tension and "positioning errors" when they do not hold parts of the organ correctly to enable the surgeon to manipulate it.

One team describes further what could go wrong: "There may be 'action too late' errors committed by the scrub nurse who does not have surgical instruments ready to hand to the surgeon as and when he/she needs them. These active errors lead to 'losses of surgical flow' where the progression of the surgical procedure is interrupted because the surgeon has to remove his/her visual focus from the heart to instruct the team."[10] Notification of the appropriate medical staff leader and documentation of the situation through whatever mechanism is available in the organization are appropriate. The right person must be available and trained to do the right activity. Staffing and training concerns are systems issues that must be addressed on a systems basis. The surgical assistant's and scrub nurse's performance in the examples above are not at the root of the failures; rather, the root causes are insufficient training and staffing.

 Do not take shortcuts, and supervise staff to ensure that they do not either. Scheduling and work load pressures encourage physicians and the entire surgical team to work as quickly and efficiently as possible. Pressures may tempt physicians to delegate procedures inappropriately to untrained or inexperienced team members. Or, attending surgeons may not be alertly hovering when needed to diagnose intraoperative complications. Proper supervision is essential when supervising residents and students, among others. Shortcuts can easily compromise patient safety.

Ensure weekend, evening, and vacation coverage by qualified colleagues. Physicians must ensure that their patients are cared for by qualified colleagues during an absence from the health care setting.

System Solution 3: Policies, Procedures, and Technology

Sentinel Event Example: Lack of Training

A surgeon requests that a new prep solution be added to the stock of solutions used during operative procedures. The prep solution's information insert indicates that the solution is flammable unless allowed to dry. The organization's OR procedures require an in-service presentation of any new product, procedure, or piece of equipment prior to use. When the surgeon asks for the solution in the OR, she is informed that although the product is available, she will not be able to use it because the nurses have not yet received training related to its use. The surgeon questions the need for a class on something as simple as a prep solution and asks for the solution. Although the nurses question the surgeon's request, they agree to it and provide the prep solution.

The circulating nurse preps the patient's neck with the new solution, and the surgeon quickly steps forward and drapes the patient. The nurse does not have the opportunity to remove the towels placed on either side of the neck to catch prep solution drippings. The

---

Sidebar 2-1. Credentialing and Privileging Basics

Credentialing is defined by the Joint Commission as "the process of obtaining, verifying, and assessing the qualifications of a health care practitioner to provide patient care services in or for a health care organization." Credentialing, or *credentials review*, as it sometimes is called, implies that an organization has specified the minimum requirements, or *credentials,* for entry into medical or other professional staff membership, for example, or for granting clinical privileges. *Credentials* are documented evidence of licensure, education, training, experience, or other qualifications. The organization determines through review of credentials whether an individual meets the requirements. Credentialing also provides information for the process of granting clinical privileges to all licensed independent practitioners in the organization.

Privileging is the process whereby a specific scope and content of patient care services (that is,

clinical privileges) are authorized for a health care practitioner by a health care organization based on evaluation of the individual's credentials and performance. When an individual is granted clinical privileges, he or she receives authorization by a health care organization to provide patient care services in or for the organization. The four activities involved in privileging are

- determining which clinical procedures or treatments the organization will offer and support;
- determining what training and experience are required for authorization to perform each clinical procedure or treatment;
- determining whether individuals applying for privileges meet these requirements and officially granting or denying requested privileges; and
- monitoring the individuals granted privileges to ensure their continued competence and practice within the scope of privileges granted.

Source: Joint Commission: *Assessing Hospital Staff Competence.* Oakbrook Terrace, IL, 2002, p 10.

presence of towels containing the pooled solution makes the situation extremely dangerous. The surgeon makes a skin incision using an electrocautery knife. The site and the drapes burst into flames. The patient suffers serious burns on the neck, chest, and face.

The surgeon and the operating staff in this example lacked the knowledge necessary to use the new product safely. They had not received the required training session, as per organization policy. More than half of the organizations experiencing sentinel events related to operative or postoperative errors reported to the Joint Commission since 1995 identified a failure to comply with policies as one root cause. Physicians, nurses, and other OR team members must be trained

and expected to follow established procedures at all times. Joint Commission "Care of the Patient" requirements address the selection of appropriate procedures, preparation of the patient for the procedures, execution of the procedures, patient monitoring, and postoperative care.

 Be knowledgeable about organizational policies and procedures. Organization leaders establish policies and procedures to reduce the risk of adverse events. The design of procedures must take into account human factors such as the tendency to take shortcuts. Policies and procedures must be available to the entire operative team so that all team members know what is expected of them.

Education about policies and procedures provides clinicians with an understanding of how the policy or procedure effectively prevents sentinel events. Leaders ensure that physicians and other team members are complying with established policies and procedures. Innovative and effective methods of communicating to physicians about policies and procedures should be developed.

 Standardize procedures across care settings. Medical staff leaders must help to ensure uniform performance of patient care processes. A collaborative, multidisciplinary approach to standardization across various settings enables collaborative learning, decreases confusion during training, and establishes consistent performance evaluation methods. For example, due to high complication rates, one organization recognized the need to standardize the procedure for inserting central-line catheters. Following implementation of a redesigned policy, consistent training, and standardized equipment, the organization significantly improved the complication rate throughout the facility. Use of standardized procedures for other high-risk activities, such as conscious sedation, emergency care, pain management, and hyperalimentation, helps to reduce the likelihood of adverse events.

 Develop and use checklists and standardized protocols whenever possible. Many industries, such as aviation, food technology, and others, have long demanded rigid adherence to well-defined protocols. The goal of such protocols is standardization. Standardization can reduce the variability of process implementation and the unneeded variety of factors that can lead to failures. For example, protocols for use of hazardous or high-alert drugs can reduce the likelihood of failures at numerous steps and linkages of steps in the medication use process. Protocols for identifying individuals at risk for falls or suicide can reduce the likelihood of failures of steps and links in the patient assessment process. The multidisciplinary,

evidence-based clinical guidelines, procedures, protocols, and algorithms developed by Mission Hospital Regional Medical Center in Mission Viejo, California, for the treatment of the organization's severe traumatic brain injury patients by trauma surgeons and other members of the trauma team reduced mortality by 27%.[11] Sidebar 2-2, page 45, describes this effort in more detail.

Protocol use makes sense in many instances. One physician-ethicist notes the following:

It is arrogant to think that each surgeon's approach to a given problem is as good as any other surgeon's approach. It is inexcusable to ignore the fact that there are documented approaches to some conditions that are demonstrated to be superior to others. In one city, early breast cancer in a certain hospital is treated most of the time by lumpectomy and radiation with lymph node sampling. Across town, it is treated 80% of the time by modified radical mastectomy with complete lymph node dissection. Among the surgeons at all hospitals, there are a variety of approaches to drains, dressings, antibiotics, and other approaches that are idiosyncratic and not subjected to objective evaluation. Is everyone correct? Our beginning efforts to develop consensus approaches are laudatory and sensible. Studies on left colon surgery demonstrate that with meticulous attention to protocol, hospitalization can be reduced to a few days, and complications and adverse events can be all but eliminated.[9]

When protocols do not currently exist, physicians can work with colleagues to create care protocols in their areas of expertise.

 Monitor consistency of compliance with procedures. Because of the critical importance of following policies and procedures, medical staff should participate in the collection and analysis of data related to compliance with policies and procedures, such as frequency of compliance with postoperative monitoring

Sidebar 2-2. Use of Guidelines and Protocols to Improve Outcomes in Patients with Severe Traumatic Brain Injury

Mission Hospital Regional Medical Center, a 271-bed acute care facility and designated trauma center for south Orange County, developed and implemented an initiative that dramatically improved the clinical outcomes of patients sustaining severe traumatic brain injury (TBI). A description of the effort follows.

For nearly two decades, the clinical outcomes of patients sustaining severe TBI at the hospital were marginal at best. Nearly half of the population expired and one-third suffered severe disability. Even though these outcomes were consistent with outcomes cited in national studies published in the 1980s, the hospital's multidisciplinary trauma team found such outcomes less than satisfactory.

In late 1995, the American Association of Neurological Surgeons (AANS) and the Brain Trauma Foundation published evidence-based clinical guidelines for managing severe TBI patients. The guidelines questioned current practices, recommended practices changes, and challenged hospitals to evaluate their care practices and examine the clinical outcomes of this high-risk group. After looking at the data, the trauma director and trauma coordinator concluded that there had to be a better way to handle TBI patients. Recommendations in the AANS guidelines represented a major paradigm shift in the management of the critically injured TBI patient. In studying the guidelines, the team quickly realized that a dramatic variance in practice existed between the guidelines and the care processes at Mission Hospital. Then-current practices, such as hyperventilation, dehydration, less than optimal blood pressure management, and the lack of means to monitor cerebral

oxygenation, were divergent from the AANS guidelines and scientific literature.

Motivated by new evidence-based national recommendations and the belief that patient outcomes could be greatly improved, in 1997 Mission Hospital's multidisciplinary trauma team began scrutinizing existing practices with TBI patients. The team examined every aspect of care for the severe TBI patient—from admission to rehabilitation, analyzing the processes and outcomes and reviewing published TBI guidelines and the scientific literature for each care process. The team then developed and refined multidisciplinary clinical guidelines, procedures, protocols, and algorithms for use with the hospital's severe TBI patients at each stage, including resuscitation in the ED, intraoperative management, and postoperative management.

Clinical outcomes for the hospital's severe TBI patients improved significantly. Historically, the severe TBI patient population incurred a high mortality and morbidity rate from injuries. Prior to the effort, 43 percent of such patients died, 30 percent survived with severe disability to persistent vegetative state, and 27 percent survived with a good outcome to moderate disability only. Within three years of undertaking the improvement project, only 16 percent of severe TBI patients died, 14 percent sustained severe disability to persistent vegetative state, and 70 percent experienced a good outcome to moderate disability. The evidence-based guidelines for severe TBI patients developed and implemented at Mission Hospital dramatically improved patient outcomes.

Source: Joint Commission: *2000 Ernest A. Codman Award* (monograph). Oakbrook Terrace, IL, 2001.

procedures, preoperative assessment, and so forth. When performance is inconsistent, managers evaluate the process to determine whether the procedure's design lends itself to compliance errors and why. Some medical and nursing directors establish a regular routine for observing the performance of specific procedures, particularly those associated with high risks.

Prevention Strategy *Use technology proven to be effective and safe.* Technological innovations can have considerable impact on patient safety and care outcomes. To ensure patient safety, physicians should be competent in the use of the latest and most advanced technology used during procedures. Health care organizations verify such competence through the credentialing and privileging process. Equipment that addresses human needs and characteristics will be most effective and must be well maintained as per organization policy. Poor equipment maintenance has been cited as a root cause of a number of operative and postoperative errors. One expert describes technical malfunctions not caused by the user as well as malfunctions caused by users.[12] The standardization of equipment and devices is critical. Users must be familiar with how to use equipment commonly required in surgical suites. Physicians can play an important role in recommending appropriate equipment to medical staff leaders.

System Solution 4: Preoperative Assessment and Postoperative Monitoring

Sentinel Event Example: Incomplete Preoperative Assessment*

A 32-year-old woman, seven months pregnant, was referred to a surgeon for treatment of "bilateral inguinal hernias." The surgeon noted, in a single line of the record, "bilateral inguinal hernias," and suggested

---

* This example appears courtesy Dwyer K: Surgery-related claims and the systems involved. *Forum* 21:1–4, summer 2001. Reprinted with permission.

hernia repair one month after the patient's planned cesarean section.

At the appointment time, the patient, who was then asymptomatic, presented to the surgeon for a preoperative exam. The brief exam did not include her groin area. Relying upon the preexisting diagnosis, the surgeon performed a herniorrhaphy, which revealed no evidence of a hernia. The postoperative course was complicated by infection and an additional procedure to remove retained suture material. The patient brought suit against the surgeon for unnecessary surgery. Her medical record was devoid of documentation of her symptoms, the physical exam, or the clinical rationale for doing the surgery.

Near-Miss Example: Faulty Monitoring

During a shoulder reduction in the ED, an obese 25-year-old man requires a considerable amount of narcotics and benzodiazepines for pain control. In the recovery period, the lack of stimulation causes a decrease in his ventilation, with a decrease in oxygen saturation. The patient is then given reversal agents for both the narcotics and benzodiazepines. Shortly thereafter, the patient is awake, alert, and has normal oxygen saturation levels.

However, the facility does not have a policy indicating how long the patient should be monitored after the use of a reversal agent, and the patient is discharged from the recovery period in the ED ten minutes later. Because the narcotics in the patient's system last longer than the reversal agent, the patient becomes renarcotized at home and is brought back to the ED by ambulance. He experiences increased sedation and an altered breathing pattern. Staff stabilize him and he is able to return home six hours later.

The lack of a complete preoperative assessment is one of the root causes associated with various operative adverse events. The events might be the result of a rush to clear a patient for surgery, missing information such as laboratory data, the existence and status of preexisting diseases not indicated in the history and physical examination (H&P), and changes in the patient's health. The lack of information might be reflected in an inappropriate choice of anesthetic or surgical procedure, the decision to use or not use a medication, or the failure to plan appropriately for the postoperative period. Examples of possible adverse events include

- failure to recognize a patient as being on anticoagulants prior to invasive procedures, resulting in bleeding;
- failure to recognize a patient as having sleep apnea, resulting in a serious respiratory response with sedation; and
- failure to identify a patient as having a medication allergy, resulting in anaphylactic reaction.

Physicians and nurses should not only observe that the preassessment is present but also review the assessment in depth to identify questionable or confusing information.

In the area of postoperative monitoring, the Joint Commission requires that patients be monitored continuously during the postoperative period. Monitoring should include

- physiological and mental status;
- status of or findings related to pathological conditions, such as drainage from incisions;
- intravenous fluids and drugs administered, including blood and blood components;
- impairments and functional status;
- pain intensity and quality, and responses to treatments; and
- unusual events or postoperative complications and their management.

Various categories of patients often come through an OR's postanesthesia care unit (PACU). Outpatients, inpatients, and same-day-admit patients should receive postoperative monitoring. Organization policies should address any differences in required monitoring. In some circumstances, a patient might be transferred directly from the OR to an intensive care unit (ICU). Leaders should consider whether the

immediate postoperative care is comparable to the PACU care and whether ICU and PACU nurses are similarly trained for immediate postoperative care. The staff member responsible for the patient's immediate postprocedural care should be identified. In the PACU, anesthesiologists are directly responsible for the patient until he or she is discharged from the recovery room. What staff member is responsible for the patient's care during the immediate postoperative period in the ICU should be clear.

Often, procedures with and without conscious sedation are done in numerous places in a facility. A consistent policy should be in place throughout a facility for postoperative monitoring in sites outside the OR's PACU. Physicians should be aware of where their patients are to be monitored and provide staff with telephone numbers at which they can be reached. In one facility, patients who had procedures completed in the endoscopy suite fell into two categories: Outpatients were transferred to the PACU for monitoring and eventual discharge, and inpatients were discharged directly to their hospital rooms. A comparison of the two groups revealed that inpatients received minimal postoperative monitoring.

 Actively involve the patient in medical decision making through the informed consent process. "The first step to addressing postoperative complications with patients takes place during the preoperative patient consent process. Conducting and documenting a discussion about potential complications heightens awareness and may minimize the surprise if something occurs," writes one expert.[5]

 Ensure that preoperative assessments are available, accurate, and complete. Nurses can help physicians guarantee that needed assessments, including the physician's H&P, are available, complete, and accurate. In addition to identifying incomplete assessment sections, the physician and nurse can also compare the information available in the assessments, laboratory reports, and various forms to ensure the consistency of data. By identifying the pieces that do not match, corrective steps can be achieved before a serious situation develops.

 Work with nursing leaders to ensure that the nursing staff knows and follows the organization's postoperative monitoring policies. The key strategy in achieving satisfactory postoperative monitoring is for the nursing staff to become familiar with postoperative monitoring policies through thorough training, orientation, and competence assessment. Collaborative efforts of the various departments, particularly the medical staff, involved in determining the postoperative monitoring policies and procedures will help ensure the identification and implementation of the best possible policies.

 Evaluate patients promptly during the postoperative period. Delays in evaluating patients, particularly those at high risk for infection and other complications, can lead to sentinel events. Increasing pain or other evidence of infection should prompt immediate evaluation. "Multiple patient complaints within a short period of time should trigger further inquiry. Although the additional visit may be inconvenient for both the clinician and the patient (post-discharge), serious complications can often be identified more quickly or avoided altogether," advises one author.[13] High-quality communication among physicians, surgeons, house staff, and nursing staff is critical.

Closing Comments

Physicians play the critical role in reducing the likelihood of sentinel events associated with operative and postoperative complications or errors. Prevention strategies address and span the breadth of challenges to safe health care. These challenges include incomplete assessment, failure to follow established policies, inadequate staff training or competence assessment, and insufficient communication or information availability. To empower physicians to make a difference, leaders must establish and maintain a collaborative environment conducive to thorough multidisciplinary communication. Patient safety excellence involves individuals, teams, and organizational policies and culture. Table 2-2, pages 49–50, summarizes key "excellence-producing" factors cited in one surgical arena. Many of these factors easily transfer to other surgical arenas.

REFERENCES

1. Leape LL, et al: The nature of adverse events in hospitalized patients: Results of the Harvard Medical Practice Study II. *NEJM* 324:377–84, Feb 1991.

2. Andrews LB, et al: An alternative strategy for studying adverse events in medical care. *Lancet* 349(9048):309–13, 1997.

3. California Medical Association: *Report of the Medical Insurance Feasibility Study.* San Francisco, 1977.

4. National Patient Safety Foundation at the American Medical Association: *Public Opinion of Patient Safety Issues: Research Findings.* Chicago, Sep 1997. Web site: www.npsf.org.

5. Dwyer K: Surgery-related claims and the systems involved. *Forum* 21:1–4, Summer 2001.

6. Joint Commission Resources: Statistics provide insight into causes of sentinel events. *Jt Comm Persp* 22:3–5, Aug 2002.

7. Joint Commission: Operative and postoperative complications: Lessons for the future. *Sentinel Event Alert* Issue 12, 4 Feb 2000.

8. Risk Management Foundation: A conversation with Lucian Leape, MD. *Forum* 21:5–7, Summer 2001, p 7.

9. Krizek TJ: Surgical error: Ethical issues of adverse events. *Arch Surg* 135:1359–66, Nov 2000.

10. Carthey J, et al: Human factors and cardiac surgery: Identifying problems and positive aspects of surgical performance. Presented at Enhancing Patient Safety and Reducing Errors in Health Care (Annenberg II), Rancho Mirage, CA, 9 Nov 1998.

11. Joint Commission: *2000 Ernest A. Codman Award* (monograph). Oakbrook Terrace, IL, 2001.

12. Hyman WA: Errors in the use of medical equipment. In Bogner MS (ed): *Human Error in Medicine.* Hillsdale, NJ: Lawrence Erlbaum Associates, 1994, p 327.

13. Rawn GL: Closed claim abstract: PA supervision in urgent care. *Forum* 19(5) Mar 1999.

Table 2-2. Excellence-Producing Factors in Pediatric Cardiac Surgery

Level	Excellence-producing factor	Definition	Practical examples
Individual level	Safety awareness	A "safety aware" surgeon expresses the attitude that every step of the procedure has to be perfect before proceeding to the next step, and he acts according to this principle.	The cardiac surgeon checks for bleed points after completing each stage of the procedure and adds extra sutures where they are needed. By doing this the surgeon reduces the likelihood that the patients will have serious post-bypass bleeding incidents.
Individual level	Self-confidence/ self-belief	The surgeon's belief in his/her ability to carry out the surgical procedure successfully. This characteristic changes over time depending on the surgeon's recent experience of the procedure.	A surgeon who has the optimum level of confidence is likely to make an appropriate surgical intervention at an appropriate time.
Individual level	Communication style	How well the surgeon communicates instructions and patient related information requests to other medical professionals.	The surgeon's communications provide the rest of the theater team with a clear framework to work in. For example, "Contact me immediately if the left arterial pressure rises above 12 and the ABP drops below 50."
Individual level	Adaptation	How well the surgeon can cope with and adapt to changes from the norm, i.e., surgical adaptation.	The surgeon adapts his/her behavior when there is an inexperienced surgical assistant. He/she issues more frequent and detailed instructions and moves the assistant's hands into the correct position.
Individual level	Cognitive flexibility	Cognitive flexibility is the ability to switch from one surgical strategy or hypothesis to another.	When diagnosing the cause(s) of post bypass ischemia, the surgeon tests the validity of a series of hypotheses and can think about multiple causes of a problem.
Individual level	Global overview	Where the surgeon's situational awareness includes all of the activity in the operating theater, not just the surgical aspects of the procedure.	The cardiac surgeon periodically requests an update on the status of the perfusion and anesthetic tasks so that he/she has an overview of what is going on in the whole of the operating theater.
Individual level	Anticipation	How well the surgeon perceives and responds to potential problems before they spiral out of control.	The cardiac surgeon quickly perceives changes in the ECG screen readings and/or the physical condition of the heart and anticipates that a major problem—e.g., myocardial infarction—may develop unless corrective action is initiated.
Individual level	Technical skill	Technical skill comprises the physical and cognitive abilities of the surgeon.	The surgeon's manual dexterity determines the speed and precision with which he/she can do the case. His/her cognitive skills, i.e., knowledge and experience of the procedure, determine the range of surgical strategies that he/she has available to use.

(continued)

Source: Carthey J, et al: Human factors and cardiac surgery: Identifying problems and positive aspects of surgical performance. Presented at Enhancing Patient Safety and Reducing Errors in Health Care (Annenberg II), Chicago, IL: National Paitent Safety Foundation,1999. Used with permission.

Table 2-2. Excellence-Producing Factors in Pediatric Cardiac Surgery (continued)

Level	Excellence-producing factor	Definition	Practical examples
Team level	Experience	The theater team's previous experience of carrying out the surgical procedure and working together.	Team stability, i.e., where the people in the team are familiar with each other's working practices enhances performance because there is better anticipation of "where the surgeon is going next."
Team level	Skill	How good the team is to carrying out their clinical tasks.	Highly skilled and experienced surgical teams have fewer "losses of surgical flow" than inexperienced surgical teams.
Team level	Redundancy	The spare resources available for use if needed.	Physical redundancy: having a second surgical assistant at the operating table. Cognitive redundancy: having spare cognitive resources in the theater team to help solve problems.
Team level	Adoption	The extent to which the team is able to cope with changes from the norm.	For example, "team adaptation": adapting to a new and inexperienced person in the theater team. An experienced surgical team member takes over the surgical tasks of an inexperienced team member if repeated "losses of surgical flow" occur.
Team level	Authority/ leadership	How well the cardiac surgeon controls activity in the operating theater.	The cardiac surgeon refuses to take messages from outside the operating theater during a case, thereby reducing the potential for "external distracters" to disrupt the theater team's tasks.
Organization	Policy	The rules that govern the way the organization does things.	An organizational policy that states that the cardiologist must try to diagnose the coronary arterial pattern of a switch patient preoperatively increases the chances that complex cardiac anatomies will be discovered preoperatively and not intra-operatively.
Organization	Planning and scheduling	The organization's philosophy and practice on how to plan clinical, research, and management activities.	Good organizational planning can reduce potential conflicts between clinical, research, and management goals. For example, organizing management meetings so that they do not overlap with the start/end of a case.
Organization	Learning mechanisms	How the organization learns from prior experience.	For example, the structure, content, and organization of death conferences (which are held following the death of a patient) will determine what is learned and who learns from a bad case.
Organization	Communication	How information is disseminated through the organization.	In organization A, the two cardiac surgeons discuss every case that has a bad outcome. This increases their learning opportunities.
Organization	Resources	The financial, human, and equipment resources that are available.	High-technology equipment like Extra Corporeal Membrane Oxygenation (ECMO) machines.
Organization	Culture	The attitudes, beliefs, and behavior of people within the organization.	Research on safety culture in other high-technology systems has shown a link between culture and safety performance.

PROTECTING PATIENTS FROM WRONG-SITE, WRONG-PERSON, OR WRONG-PROCEDURE SURGERY

O f all the failures that occur in health care settings, one of the most disturbing is perhaps wrong-site, wrong-person, or wrong-procedure surgery. A surgeon amputates the wrong leg. An invasive cardiac electrophysiology study is performed on the wrong patient. A mastectomy is performed on a patient who should have had a lumpectomy. These failures should be 100% preventable, yet they occur in reputable health care organizations with well-trained and well-intentioned health care teams. They occur relatively infrequently, but when they do occur, their effects can devastate patients and care providers alike.

Cause for Concern

Data from the Joint Commission's sentinel event database, including more than 1,600 sentinel events reviewed by the organization from January 1995 through May 2002, indicate that wrong-site, wrong-person, or wrong-procedure surgery have accounted for 11.2% of all sentinel events, making this the third most frequently identified type of event. Although most of the errors involve the laterality aspects of operating on the wrong side, there have also been situations where the wrong procedure was done at the correct site or the correct procedure was done on the wrong patient. As of May 2002, 184 cases had been reviewed by the Joint Commission. These may represent only a small portion of the actual total events because significant underreporting is likely. It is important to note that wrong-site, wrong-person, or wrong-procedure surgery failures are actually a subset of surgical complications. If all

three categories of sentinel events were added together, the umbrella category would constitute the most frequent category of sentinel event, by far.

No specialty or care setting can consider itself immune to the problem. Earlier data analysis based on 126 cases indicated that

- 41% were related to orthopedic/podiatric surgery;
- 20% were related to general surgery;
- 14% were related to neurosurgery;
- 11% were related to urologic surgery; and
- the remaining 14% were related to dental/oral maxillofacial, cardiovascular-thoracic, ear-nose-throat, and ophthalmologic surgery.[1]

Of the 58% of the cases that occurred in either a hospital-based ambulatory surgery unit or a freestanding ambulatory setting, 29% occurred in the inpatient OR and 13% in other inpatient sites such as the ED or ICU. Seventy-six percent involved surgery on the wrong body part or site, 13% involved surgery on the wrong patient, and 11% involved the wrong surgical procedure.

Data from professional organizations are equally dramatic. For example, the American Academy of Orthopaedic Surgeons (AAOS) reported that during a 35-year career, an orthopedic surgeon has a one in four chance of performing a wrong-site surgery.[2] The organization also reported that during an 11-year period ending in 1995, 225 orthopedic wrong-site surgery claims were filed through 22 different physician insurance companies nationwide. Most orthopedic errors occurred during arthroscopy and usually involved surgeons performing the correct procedure but on the wrong side. From 1979 to 2000, the Pennsylvania Medical Society Insurance Company paid out millions in claims for 88 cases of wrong-site surgery involving such varied specialties as orthopedics, ophthalmology, neurosurgery, urology, and interventional radiology.[3]

Professional organizations, associations, and regulatory bodies are actively addressing the problem. Despite their efforts, wrong-site, wrong-person, or wrong-procedure surgery remains a significant concern across the United States. In February 1997 the AAOS issued a revised *Advisory Statement* highlighting recommendations and methods for eliminating wrong-site surgery, as well as the appropriate management following the discovery of wrong-site surgery.[4] "Although the wrong-site surgery problem has been addressed on a local level in many areas of the country, there has been no organized national effort to eliminate wrong-site surgery," says S. Terry Canale, MD, past president of the AAOS.[5] "The American Academy of Orthopaedic Surgeons believes that a unified effort among surgeons, hospitals, and other health care providers to initiate preoperative and other institutional regulations can effectively eliminate wrong-site surgery in the United States. The AAOS urges other surgical and health care practitioner groups to join the effort in implementing effective controls to eliminate this system problem."[5]

In February 2001, the New York State Department of Health released the final report of its Preoperative Protocols Panel, outlining steps for preventing wrong-site surgery, wrong procedures, and procedures on the wrong patient (shown later in this chapter, in Sidebar 3-3).[6] The guidelines, applicable to all settings, are considered baselines that hospitals, surgery centers, and practitioners can build upon and tailor to their settings. Shared with all New York State hospitals and ambulatory care centers, the guidelines emphasize enhanced communication among surgical team members, and three independent verifications,

including marking or identifying the correct site, and having the surgeon see and speak with the patient in the perioperative area.

Clearly, the public will no longer tolerate injuries involving wrong-site, wrong-person, or wrong-procedure surgery and is influencing action through state agencies and other regulatory bodies. In June 2001 in Florida, the Board of Medicine instituted stiff penalties for physicians and organizations involved in wrong-site surgery. Penalties for physicians now include fines up to $10,000, 5 hours of risk management education, 50 hours of community service, and a 1-hour lecture to the medical community on wrong-site surgery.

The Physician's Role

Traditionally, surgeons have had primary responsibility for ensuring that the correct patient and correct site are being treated and that the correct procedure is being performed. However, root cause analyses of multiple wrong-site, wrong-person, or wrong-procedure cases demonstrate convincingly that multidisciplinary patient assessment and preparation; verification of the correct site, patient, and procedure in the OR; and communication among caregivers are the most critical functions and, therefore, the locus of effective strategies for reducing the risk of wrong-site, wrong-person, or wrong-procedure failures.

At the most fundamental level, every physician and surgical team member needs to recognize that such failures could happen. "It's not a common problem in the statistical scheme of things. I've been operating successfully for 12 years and I don't know of any colleagues who have operated on the wrong site either. However, that's not to say that I can't see how slipups could occur at a good practice, with a competent doctor," notes one surgeon.[7] Physicians need to maintain a high degree of awareness of the possibility of this type of failure.

All caregivers (including surgeons, anesthesiologists, and nurses) should be involved in checking the identity of the patient and the correctness of the surgical site and procedure before beginning a surgical procedure. Surgeons, anesthesiologists, and nurses take numerous precautions to prevent wrong-site, wrong-person, or wrong-procedure surgery. But at times even these measures have not prevented failures. The cooperation and interdependence of all health care staff members working as equal members of a team are required to help prevent wrong-site, wrong-person, or wrong-procedure sentinel events.

Common Systems Failures

The causes of wrong-site, wrong-person, or wrong-procedure sentinel events cross disciplinary boundaries and, like all other types of sentinel events, reflect systems failures. Contributing environmental factors cited by two authors include increasing subspecialization, reduced staffing, and pressure to reduce lengths of stay.[8] "These forces act on all hospitals to reduce the likelihood that an individual patient will be surrounded by physicians and nurses who know her [or him] well, understand why she [he] is hospitalized, and actively coordinate planned tests and treatments. They act synergistically to increase the probability that the wrong patient will undergo an invasive procedure [or the right patient will undergo the wrong procedure or the right procedure at the wrong site]," comment two authors.[8]

JCAHO has identified several factors that contribute to the risk of such a sentinel event (the percentages reflect occurrence in the cases reviewed)[9]:
• Emergency cases (19%);
• Unusual patient characteristics such as physical deformity or massive obesity that might alter the usual process for equipment setup or positioning of the patient (16%);
• Unusual time pressures to start or complete the procedure (13%);
• Unusual equipment or setup in the OR (13%);
• Multiple surgeons involved in the case (13%); and
• Multiple procedures being performed during a single surgical visit (10%).

JCAHO's sentinel event database identifies root cause, systems-oriented failure sources. The root causes identified by the hospitals usually involved more than one factor; however, the majority involved breakdowns in communication among surgical team members or between surgical team members and the patient and family. Other contributing causes included policy issues, such as marking of the surgical site was not required; verification in the OR and a verification checklist were not required; and patient assessment was incomplete, including an incomplete preoperative assessment. Staffing issues, distraction factors, availability of pertinent information in the OR, and organizational cultural issues were also cited as contributing risk factors.

Figure 3-1, page 54, illustrates the percentage of wrong-site, wrong-person, or wrong-procedure failures attributed to each root cause. For most failures, multiple causes were identified. A thorough look at the root causes and responsibilities of physicians as team members is critical to the successful development and implementation of effective failure prevention strategies. The remainder of this chapter focuses on prevention strategies physicians can use when working within a team environment to help reduce the likelihood of wrong-site, wrong-person, or wrong-procedure sentinel events.

System Solution 1: Communication

Sentinel Event Example: Communication Failure Among Caregiving Staff

A review of a medical record by nursing staff indicates that a patient's H&P was completed by the patient's internist. The H&P notes that the patient has bilateral arthritis of both knees. The H&P concludes that the patient is scheduled for a total knee replacement, but there is no indication of which knee. The surgeon has no preoperative notes in the record because the patient had been admitted the day of the surgery. Because the

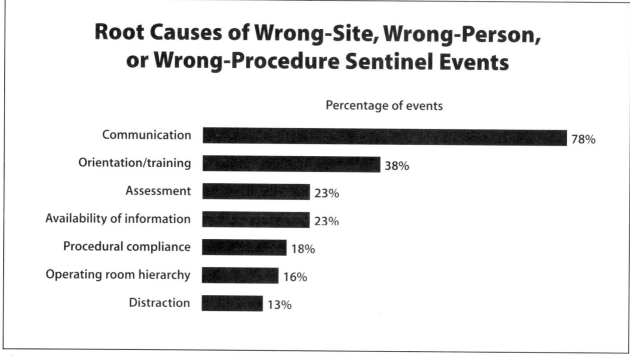

Figure 3-1. This chart illustrates the percentage of wrong-site, wrong-person, or wrong-procedure sentinel events attributed to each root cause for events reviewed by the Joint Commission between January 1995 and May 2002. For most failures, multiple causes were identified.

patient does not speak English well, the nursing staff completes the informed consent based solely on information noted in the OR schedule, which calls for a right-side total knee replacement. The surgery is performed on the wrong knee.

Near Miss Example: Failure to Communicate Effectively with Patient and Family

A surgeon's office staff mails informed consent forms to patients. Patients are instructed to sign the consent form and bring it to the hospital the day of surgery. An elderly patient receives the informed consent for a "cervical laminectomy with fusion." The woman does not recall the surgeon's mention of fusion. She calls her son, who had accompanied her during the office visit when the surgery was discussed. The son, who is a physician, explains that not only was the "fusion" part wrong, but the procedure was to be a "lumbar laminectomy"—at the other end of the back. The woman communicates the error to the physician's office, and office staff provide corrected information.

As illustrated by these examples, communication issues fall into two categories: communication among staff members and communication with patient/family.

 Communicate with staff and encourage open and direct communication from staff. Inaccurate or incomplete communication among caregivers increases the risk of adverse events. At times, wrong-site, wrong-person, or wrong-procedure failures have occurred because certain members of the team are excluded from participation in the process for site, procedure, or person verification or are hesitant to point out possible errors due to an intensely hierarchical culture. If the verification process relies solely on the surgeon's involvement, do staff feel free to question his or her decision?

Physicians must communicate with staff in a manner that encourages teamwork and open communication. The American College of Surgeons stresses the importance of teamwork in any surgical situation. "It is most important that there be cooperative openness between the surgeon and the nurses," says Tom Russell, MD, executive director, American College of Surgeons.[1] "The two groups must both take responsibility, and if there are questions, they should stop and clarify to be sure everyone is on the same page. No one should make assumptions."[1] With increased awareness of risk of wrong-site, wrong-person, or wrong-procedure sentinel events, professionals must speak up and encourage all members of the surgical team to do so as well.

Documentation in records is essential, but verbal communication helps to enhance information transfer. An OR nurse should receive a report from the nurse caring for a patient, review relevant documentation, verify the information with the patient, and document the findings. In the OR, the surgical team must be informed of the site of the procedure and participate in the verification process. Total reliance on the surgeon for verifying the site and procedure is problematic. In the office, clinic, or extended care facility, the patient's assessment and informed consent should be processed with pertinent details that indicate the exact site of the procedure. In a teaching hospital, the house staff should be an integral piece of the communication loop. The method for communicating this information should be part of a formal, structured process.

Important risk reduction strategies related to team communication recommended by JCAHO include the following[1]:
- Obtain oral verification of the patient, surgical site, and procedure in the OR by each member of the surgical team. The physician can initiate this verification process, or it can be initiated by a member of the nursing staff. The process should not be rushed, and if anyone expresses a concern, it should be addressed thoroughly before further steps are taken to proceed with the surgery.
- Surgical teams should consider taking a "time out" in the OR to verify the correct patient,

site, and procedure, using active—not passive—communication techniques. For example, the surgeon could ask each team member to state the operative site, indicating the proper laterality.

Prevention Strategy | *Engage the patient (or family, when appropriate) in identifying the correct surgical site and procedure.* It is important to thoroughly complete the informed consent process. The informed consent process is designed to involve the patient and family as full participants in care decisions. When it is performed well, it should protect the patient and physician from wrong-site, wrong-person, and wrong-procedure sentinel events. In practice, however, as described in the examples in this section, the process is often deeply flawed. Commenting on informed consent in teaching hospitals, two authors note:

> Obtaining consent is frequently delegated to an overburdened or exhausted physician who has not met the patient previously and does not know the details of the medical history. Cultural or social barriers to effective communication may be neither appreciated nor overcome. Although expected benefits and risks may be briefly described, truly involving the patient in the decision-making process is often not a top priority. Patients frequently cannot recall crucial information about procedures within hours of giving consent.[8]

Failure to involve the patient or family, where appropriate, in the process of identifying the correct site or procedure through the informed consent process can result in a wrong-site or wrong-procedure sentinel event. Many informed consent policies and procedures are elaborate but fraught with pitfalls. Handling informed consent through the mail is one such process. As evident in the sentinel event example, completing the informed consent document without proper information in hand presents enormous error risk. When the surgeon obtains only verbal informed consent during discussions with the patient and family, for example, nursing staff are totally dependent on possibly erroneous information with which to complete consent forms.

Joint Commission requirements regarding informed consent are outlined in the "Patient Rights and Organization Ethics" and "Care of Patients" chapters of the accreditation manuals. Informed consent must be obtained, and before it is obtained for operative and other procedures, the risks, benefits, and potential complications associated with procedures must be discussed with the patient and family.

JCAHO advises patients and family members to make sure that there is total agreement among themselves, their primary care physician, and the surgeon about exactly what will be done and where. JCAHO also recommends that patients ask their surgeon to have the surgical site marked with a permanent marker and to be involved in marking the site.[10] Physicians can encourage patients and families to assume a more proactive role in their care.

 Avoid using abbreviations when communicating about surgical sites and procedures. Spelling out left and right and the names of operative procedures helps to reduce confusion and the opportunity for error. All health care professionals must ensure legibility of information entered on patient charts. Use of acronyms that may not be known by all health care team members should be avoided.

System Solution 2: Verification Process and Availability of Information

Near-Miss Example: Faulty Operative Site Verification Process

A review of a postoperative medical record for a patient who had a craniotomy for a temporal lesion reveals that no preoperative identification of the side of the lesion took place. No site verification information is included in the H&P, the nursing assessment, the anesthesiology

assessment, or the physician's progress notes. The informed consent lists only "temporal craniotomy." The only mention of the lesion site (left versus right) appears on one radiology report. The organization has no operative site verification process. Only the surgeon verifies the site in the OR. The physician performs surgery on the correct side of the brain, but a wrong-site surgery error could easily have occurred.

Near-Miss Example: Patient Verification

Two outpatient surgery patients are sitting in the waiting area prior to having the same procedure on different limbs. The first name of one patient, "Morris," coincidentally is the same as the last name of the other patient. When the nurse enters the waiting area and call, "Morris," the wrong patient follows the nurse to the wrong OR. Fortunately, the nurse is trained to also ask for a birth date and Social Security number before applying an identification wristband. The nurse identifies the error.

Sentinel Event Example: Failed Operative Site Verification Process

A nurse verifies with a male patient that his arthroscopic surgery is for the right knee. This correlates with the posting and the consent form. The surgeon talks with the patient in the holding area and places a dot above the patient's left knee, thereby marking the wrong knee. Neither the nurse nor the surgeon communicate in the OR about the procedure site. The surgeon operates on the wrong knee of the now anesthetized patient.

These examples illustrate the importance of a thorough verification process to guarantee that the correct patient is matched with the correct procedure and that the correct operative site is identified. Such processes are often flawed because of the absence of one or more factors, including
- a formal procedure;
- involvement of the patient in the verification procedure;
- a final check in the OR;
- oral communication in the verification process;

- relevant information in the OR; and
- a checklist to guarantee that all information has been reviewed.[1]

The wrong-site surgery in the third example could have been prevented if a step in the verification procedures required pre-incision verification of the correct site by each team member. The verification technique should require oral verification of the correct site in the OR by each member of the team. Table 3-1, right, provides a list of people who should participate in and items that can be used in the verification process.

In some instances reviewed by the Joint Commission and reported in the literature, the wrong procedure was performed at the correct site. This sentinel event reflects a failure to verify the procedure, perhaps as a result of the lack of adequate information in the OR. An exacting but workable policy regarding the identification of the procedure and site of surgery requires a multidisciplinary, collaborative effort in which physicians should be integrally involved. From the initial scheduling of the procedure to its actual performance, multiple people should be involved in this complex endeavor.

 Take part in creating an organizationwide preoperative verification process, such as a checklist, to confirm that appropriate documents are available. The availability of critical information in the OR is a must. Physician leaders play an active role in developing and implementing a thorough preoperative verification process to ensure that all needed information is in hospital and ambulatory surgery facility ORs. As described in the Introduction, use of a preoperative verification process is one of the JCAHO National Patient Safety Goals and Recommendations for 2003.

The necessary components of verification and documents that are listed on a preoperative verification checklist include
- direct observation of the marked operative site; and

Table 3-1. People and Items Helpful to the Verification Process

People who can verify the surgical site:
- Surgeon
- Anesthesiologist and/or certified registered nurse anesthetist
- RN on the nursing unit
- RN in the preoperative holding area
- Circulating RN
- Patient and/or family

Documentation that can be used to verify the surgical site:
- Procedure schedule
- Operative consent
- History and physical
- Nursing assessment
- Preanesthesia assessment
- X-ray films and reports
- Surgeon's office notes
- A mark on the site
- Site checklist

Some of these people or items may not apply in every case. Each organization should determine consistent elements in the verification process.

- all documents referencing the intended operative procedure and site, including
  - the clinical record,
  - x-rays and other imaging studies and their reports,
  - the informed consent document,
  - the OR schedule and record, and
  - the anesthesia preassessment record.

A description of a thorough checklist system used by some organizations appears in Sidebar 3-1, page 58. A sample checklist developed by one health care organization appears in Figure 3-2, page 59.

Two steps are frequently missing from checklist use. The first step is reviewing the information in reports and assessments for content. This obviously goes beyond simply noting the presence of the various reports and assessments. The second step involves ensuring agreement from all team members about the information collected and not simply checking the information independently.

One strategy suggested by experts to help reduce the likelihood of an error involving the wrong procedure performed at the correct site is for the nurse to place the patient's chart on a stand in the OR and open it to the surgeon's notes describing the planned procedure. The surgeon could then quickly review the record prior to beginning. Surgeons can ask nursing staff to help ensure the use and availability of critical information in the OR, for example, by helping make notes available to the surgeon.

 Verify the proper patient, procedure, and surgical site, following the organization's protocols for doing so. Obtain oral verification of the patient, surgical site, and procedure in the OR from every member of the surgical team. Implement the organizationwide process to mark the surgical site, and involve the patient in the marking process. The surgical team should confirm the signature site. Consistent use of uniform organizationwide systems for verifying the patient, procedure, and surgical site, and specifically for marking the surgical site, help reduce the risk of wrong-site, wrong-procedure, and wrong-patient surgery. Figure 3-3, page 60, provides a sample policy and procedure for identification of operative sites.

Leaders must determine who is to mark the site, when the site is to be marked, and how the site is to be marked. The policy for marking the site must be precise and consistent, or the marking is useless and possibly dangerous. If one physician uses an *X* to indicate the site, but another surgeon uses *X* to denote "not the site," then the process is fraught with peril.

Sidebar 3-1. Description of a Verification Checklist

Some facilities have developed a verification checklist that includes both the documents and the personnel involved in the case. The form has three columns: the components being checked, a column titled *RIGHT,* and column titled *LEFT.* The person examining a document initials the correct box, indicating the side recorded in the document. A person marking the site or questioning the patient initials the appropriate box. Each health care provider marks the site he or she has discussed with the patient. The checklist can be started by anyone, at any point in the process. Finally, in the OR, the circulating nurse checks for any items not addressed, documents that all the initialed boxes are in the same column, and announces to the surgeon the site indicated by the checklist. If any initialed box is not consistent with the other boxes, the process is halted until the situation is clarified. Discrepancies in the checklist are readily apparent.

In 1997 the AAOS published an advisory statement on wrong-site surgery, that formed the basis of its subsequent "Sign Your Site" educational program for orthopedic surgeons.[4] The AAOS recommended a protocol for orthopedic surgeons to prevent even one more incident of wrong-site surgery. The protocol called for

- a review of the operative procedure with the patient and OR personnel prior to surgery;
- a review of the patient's chart in the OR prior to surgery;
- the surgeon to initial the operative site in a manner that cannot be overlooked, using a permanent marking pen and in a manner that will clearly be incorrect if transferred onto another body area prior to surgery; and
- the surgeon to operate through or adjacent to the initialed site. Surgeons should not proceed unless the signature is visible.

Preoperative Verification Checklist

Table 1

Preoperative Verification Checklist

Procedure _____ Date _____ Time _____ Date stamp _____

Initial each line when verified or completed. Write "not applicable (n/a)" for those items that are not applicable.

Preoperative verification checklist:

Initial	Initial	Verification of the presence	Comments
____	____	Patient understanding confirms physicians order	
____	____	Schedule coincides with physician's order for site/sided procedure	
____	____	Physician's order matches consent*	
____	____	Patient and/or family member verbalization coincides with consent*	
____	____	Diagnostic reports present coincide with site/side (specify)*	
____	____	Site marked by ___ patient ___ family member ___ other _____	

Initial	Initial	Verification of the presence	Comments
____	____	General consent for treatment (completed and signed)	
____	____	Consents for procedure (completed and signed)	
____	____	Blood consent (need for type and cross-match or type and screen) or refusal	
____	____	Sterilization consent (if applicable)	
____	____	Other consents: _____	
____	____	Identification band on*	
____	____	History and physical examination repeat	

Initial	Initial	Verification of the presence	Comments
____	____	Allergy profile completed and in chart	
____	____	Laboratory results reviewed and in chart; abnormal results reported to: _____	
____	____	Electrocardiogram results reviewed and in chart; abnormal results reported to: _____	
____	____	Preoperative medications given	
____	____	Patient profile, patient care summary, and graphics completed on chart	
____	____	NPO (nothing by mouth) since _____	
____	____	Last void at _____	
____	____	Preps completed _____	
____	____	Antiembolism devices on (if ordered)	
____	____	Loose teeth? no ____ yes ____ specify _____	

Unresolved/outstanding issues: _____

Valuables checklist:	None	Removed	To procedure	Given to
Orthodontic appliances/dentures	____	____	_____	_____
Eye glasses	____	____	_____	_____
Contacts ___ right ___ left	____	____	_____	_____
Prosthesis	____	____	_____	_____
Jewelry/earrings	____	____	_____	_____
Hearing aids ___ right ___ left	____	____	_____	_____
Other: _____	____	____	_____	_____

To procedure at _____ via _____

Signature/time   Initials   Signature/time   Initials   Signatures/time   Initials

*Indicates this must be verified by two RNs.

(*Adapted from* Pre-Procedure Verification Checklist *[2000], with permission from Spectrum Health, Grand Rapids, Mich*)

Figure 3-2. This checklist outlines a logical, sequential series of events to ensure correctness and completeness of a patient's preparation for surgery. Redundancy is built into the checklist by requiring two clinical staff members to check certain steps.

Source: Brown B, Riippa M, Shaneberger K: Promoting patient safety through preoperative patient verification. *AORN J* 74(5):690–8. Nov 2001. Used with permission.

Identification of Operative Site
Policy and Procedure

Administrative   X
Clinical   _____

Policy

- The side and site of all procedures will be documented in the physician's orders, on the consent for surgery form, and in the completed history and physical.
- When the surgery necessitates identification of right from left the surgeon and the patient together will identify and mark the surgical site before entering the OR.
- When procedures (for example, urology, orthopedics) require image studies to determine the operative site, the procedure must not commence until the surgeon has verified the image studies and the site.

Purpose

- To prevent errors and injuries to the surgical patient.
- To ensure the accuracy of the proposed surgical procedure as indicated on the consent for operation and anesthesia.
- To identify the right or left side, when applicable.

Procedure

- The surgery scheduling clerk
  - identifies the side and site when the procedure is scheduled.
- The preoperative RN does the following:
  - verifies procedure and site by checking the chart for documentation and comparing information with patient's understanding of impending surgical procedure; and
  - checks the chart for documentation and compares information using the
    - history and physical;
    - consent form;
    - physician's orders;
    - physician's progress notes;
    - posted surgical schedule; and
    - patient's verbal verification of side and or site.
  - documents verification of procedure site on nursing documentation record.

- If the documentation does not indicate the appropriate site, the patient will remain in the ambulatory care unit or preoperative area until the surgeon is contacted and identifies the correct procedure site.
- The circulating nurse
  - verifies patient and procedure site using first two bullets under the preoperative RN.
- The surgeon or patient does the following:
  - documents the designated procedure site on the consent for operations and anesthesia form,
  - documents the designated procedure site in the patient's preoperative progress notes, and
  - includes the operative procedure site identification in the history and physical.
- Together the surgeon and patient identify the surgical site and place a mark near the site of the incision, if the surgery requires identification of right from left. Locate the mark so it is visible after surgical drapes are placed, and document this on the preoperative record.
- The circulating nurse verifies the above information and the presence of the mark, if applicable, before the patient is taken into the OR.
- The anesthesia care provider verifies the consent and confirms the correct procedure and site before sedating the patient.
- The patient will not be draped until the team confirms the type of surgery and visually identifies the marked surgical site, if applicable.
- The surgeon will arrange imaging studies for viewing and confirm that they belong to the correct patient.
- Before making a skin incision, the surgeon will confirm imaging studies and check for the marked surgical site. There will be verbal communication among all members of the surgical team confirming the correct procedure and the correct site before starting surgery. This will be documented in the OR and anesthesia records.
- Before opening any prosthesis, the size and name of the prosthesis will be verbally stated by the surgeon, the scrub person, and the circulating nurse. The circulating nurse will show the box, when possible, to the scrub person for additional verification.

Figure 3-3. This policy and procedure outlines the tasks performed by each member of the surgical team to ensure the correct identification of the surgical site.

Reprinted with permission, *SSM™*, Dec 2001, p 54. Copyright © AORN, Inc, 2170 S Parker Road, Suite 300, Denver, CO 80231.

Some experts recommend using a purple indelible pen that will be visible on all skin tones.[7] The AAOS recommends using a permanent surgical pen, which can be sterile or unsterile. These marks usually last five to seven days and are not believed to have an effect on infection rates.[11] One organization that experienced physician noncompliance with site marking found that its policy was not being followed because the marking ink was upsetting to patients, especially those with breast cancer. "Taking into account the emotional issues of patient illness, especially breast cancer, discussion now occurs with the patient before marking ink is used. Patients are educated on and made part of the process, and they understand that it is critical to their safety," describes one writer.[12]

To prevent spinal surgery at the wrong level site, AAOS recommends the surgeon's use of markers that do not move and double-checking the level of the spine with an intraoperative x-ray that marks the exact vertebral level of surgery. Following the review of 11 closed claims involving spine surgery performed at the wrong level, the Midwest Medical Insurance Company of Minneapolis, Minnesota, issued a risk management advisory in February 1997, recommending the following to surgeons[13]:
- Review all necessary documents that indicate what levels are to be operated on.
- Use a reliable technique to identify the level:
  – Expose the lamina at the operative site;
  – Mark the intended level using an instrument or clip at the level of the exposed laminae;
  – X-ray the patient and personally interpret the x-ray; and
  – Indelibly mark the site by cautery, stitch, or "bone bite" before moving the x-ray marker.
- Work with radiologists to develop consistent level terminology (for example, "L3-4," not "L-3") and consistent conventions for counting and labeling vertebrae.

A revised report issued by the AAOS in 1998 noted that the simple use of an *X* to identify the correct or incorrect site or side had not been consistently

successful.[14] Other contributing causes cited for wrong-site surgery included the surgeon not being present in the OR for induction of anesthesia or preoperative preparation of the patient and the surgeon frequently being "rushed," and the prone or lateral positioning of the patient being disorienting for the surgeon.

Any surgeon or organization that currently uses an *X* as a site marker or a *yes* and *no* marking system should consider the following[7]:
- Marking *no* on the wrong side can be mistaken for *on* when viewed from the other side.
- Marking the nonsurgical limb with the word *no* is not useful because the nonsurgical limb is likely to not be visible when the patient is draped.
- As mentioned earlier, *X* marks have created confusion regarding whether *X* means it is the correct side or the wrong side. Does an *X* signify "*X* marks the spot," or "not here"?
- Initials on the surgical site cannot be mistaken.

After two years of educational efforts, the AAOS estimates that approximately 60% of its members were following its Sign Your Site protocol. Says Canale, past president of the AAOS, "The only real obstacles are those surgeons who say they are too busy to double-check."[7] Canale notes that there are three very basic checks that, if followed consistently, can help to eliminate the risk of a wrong-site surgery. "First of all, don't operate if the site isn't signed. Secondly, mark the radiographs of the operative sight with 'left' or 'right' to eliminate the potential for a reverse image. Lastly, check the patient consent form, which should always specify the site and procedure."[7] Because internal sites (such as an intestinal polyp), cannot be marked, verbal communication is vital.

Patients with the same name or similar-sounding names present a particular challenge. The most important strategy for preventing a sentinel event involving wrong-patient surgery is to develop and implement a standardized protocol to verify patient identity. Computerized verification systems, such as bar coding, can help to reduce system failures. "A particular team member must be charged with matching the bar code on the patient's identity bracelet to the bar code on the medication, blood product, or invasive procedure schedule," note two experts.[8] Physicians must be part of the team that verifies that the correct patient is being operated on *before* an incision is made.

 Help ensure that staff understand the verification policy and process. Several nurses are usually involved in preparing the patient for surgery. Responsibilities may vary considerably, but everyone involved must understand the process for identifying the correct surgical site. Staffing levels and staff orientation, training, and competence assessment play a major role in root causes of wrong-site, wrong-procedure, and wrong-patient surgery. Organization leaders must ensure that enough personnel have proper orientation and training to follow the established policies and procedures. Staff must be properly trained in the appropriate verification techniques and must be able to recognize unacceptable practices. Staff competence in verification policies and procedures must be evaluated on a regular basis. Physicians should alert medical staff leaders to situations in which staff competence or staffing levels could place a patient at risk for wrong-site, wrong-procedure, or wrong-patient surgery.

System Solution 3: Patient Assessment

Sentinel Event Example: Poor Communication

An elderly patient arrives for a carpal tunnel procedure. The patient's escort is asked to remain in the waiting area. Unfortunately, the H&P does not indicate that the patient has some subtle memory problems, and a mental evaluation is not part of the nurse's evaluation. The surgery schedule has the wrong wrist specified for the surgery. The always-agreeing patient responds "Yes" to the nurse's question "So we're performing the surgery on your left wrist, is that correct?" The operation is performed on the wrong limb because no other member of the surgical team confirms operative site.

Rather than tell the patient the specific site, it is often useful to ask the question in a manner that requires the patient to state the site (that is, "Which hand are we operating on today?"). The lack of a thorough preoperative assessment or H&P of the patient is a frequent contributing factor to wrong-site surgery. Often, failure to review the medical record or imaging studies in the immediate preoperative period is involved. The site of the surgery and the surgical procedure must be clearly noted in the assessment. A "total knee replacement" statement in the chart does not indicate the side of the procedure. Laterality is a crucial element in describing the surgical site.

 Identify the surgical site and procedure in the H&P and help ensure its identification in the preoperative assessment.

Physicians are responsible for complete and accurate H&Ps. A note that merely indicates "H&P dictated" is not a useful document. In one case, a surgeon felt that he could submit the same H&P that he had used for the patient three weeks earlier when the patient had a different procedure. Obviously, if the surgeon does not update the findings, the listed procedure will be wrong and therefore useless in verifying the procedure site.

Closing Comments

Physicians play a leadership role in the prevention of wrong-site, wrong-person, or wrong-procedure failures. As leaders of the OR team, they establish the culture of communication, multidisciplinary collaboration, and vigilant adherence to procedures and protocols established to help reduce the likelihood of wrong-site, wrong-person, or wrong-procedure surgery. Failure reduction strategies must focus on communication, teamwork, procedural compliance, and accurate assessment. Sidebars 3-2 through 3-4, pages 63–64, summarize strategies spanning these areas that are recommended by a pediatric surgeon, JCAHO, and the New York State Health Department.

Sidebar 3-2. A Surgeon's Advice on Preventing Wrong-Site Surgery

Paul A. Brisson, MD, a pediatric surgeon practicing in upstate New York, recommends to colleagues the following:

1. Fill out your own consent form while you're with the patient in the examining room to assure the correct site is noted.

2. Dictate or write the H&P *immediately* after seeing the patient, while the details are still fresh. Don't stack your charts and dictate them at the end of the day, particularly when location is critical. Have a copy sent to the hospital so that it's in the patient's chart at the time of surgery.

3. Talk to the patient in the holding [or preoperative] area. Confirm the operation with the patient and family. Remember that many patients neither know nor understand what operation they're having. A mark can be placed on the surgical site at this time.

4. Be sure the consent matches the OR schedule.

5. If the operation involves X-rays, see that the films are in the OR and are correctly labeled. Check that the patient's name is the same as the name on the *film* (not the folder).

6. Before starting the operation, review your notes.

7. Prep and drape the surgical site *yourself*.

8. Limit distracting small talk and phone calls in the OR.

9. When preparing to operate on an infant's hernia, have the parent physically touch the location of the hernia to avoid confusion.

10. Above all, start the day expecting big mistakes to be made.

Source: Brisson PA: Right side—or left? How to avoid this malpractice nightmare. *Medical Economics*. 19:12–3, Feb 1999. Used with permission.

Sidebar 3-3. JCAHO Recommendations for the Prevention of Wrong-Site, Wrong-Person, or Wrong-Procedure Sentinel Events

• Clearly mark the operative site and involve the patient in the marking process to enhance the reliability of the process.

• Require an oral verification of the correct site in the OR by each member of the surgical team.

• Develop a verification checklist that includes all documents referencing the intended operative procedure and site, including the medical record, x-rays, and other imaging studies and their reports; the informed consent document, the OR record, and the anesthesia record; and direct observation of the marked operative site on the patient.

• Ensure personal involvement of the surgeon in obtaining informed consent.

• Consider taking a "time out" in the OR to verify the correct patient, procedure, and site, using active—not passive—communication techniques.

• Ensure through ongoing monitoring that verification procedures are followed for high-risk procedures.

Sources: Joint Commission: A follow-up review of wrong site surgery. *Sentinel Event Alert* Issue 24, 5 Dec 2001. Joint Commission: Lessons learned: Wrong site surgery. *Sentinel Event Alert* Issue 6, 28 Aug 1998.

Sidebar 3-4. New York State Health Department Recommendations for the Prevention of Wrong-Site, Wrong-Person, or Wrong-Procedure Sentinel Events

The Commission of the New York State Health Department adopted these recommendations as a standard of care for hospitals to ensure safe patient care outcomes and avoid surgical errors in a variety of patient care settings:

- Hospitals should develop and implement policies and procedures to assure there are at least three independent verifications of the surgical site, location, and correct patient identification.
- The attending physician should sign the consent form prior to the induction of anesthesia, confirming the accuracy of the document, including the description of the procedure.
- As one of the three independent verifications, it is recommended that the surgeon of record mark or unequivocally identify the site and/or side prior to surgery. The marking technique should be determined by the facility.
- Whenever possible, the surgeon of record or his/her designee should physically see and talk to the patient in the perioperative area on the day of surgery.
- When laterality (the procedure is specific to one side of the body) is at issue, the words should be spelled out in their entirety, on the operative schedule and the operative consent form.
- The anticipated level(s) for spinal surgery should be indicated on the operative schedule and the operative consent form. Levels may be modified later if operative findings indicate differences.
- For OR settings (for other settings, use appropriate personnel), the circulating nurse will ensure:
  - the correct patient is present;
  - the consent has been signed by the surgeon of record on the day of surgery;
  - the appropriate surgical side/site has been identified/marked;
  - the surgeon has selected for display appropriate and relevant radiological films for the planned procedure (the surgeon of record determines what is appropriate and relevant); and
  - there is agreement as to the planned procedure, which has been verified with the surgeon, anesthesia personnel, and circulating nurses. The agreement must be documented in the medical record.

Source: New York State Health Department releases pre-operative protocols to enhance safe surgical care. Web site: www.health.state.ny.us/nysdoh/commish/2001/preop.htm. Used with permission.

REFERENCES

1. Joint Commission: A follow-up review of wrong site surgery. *Sentinel Event Alert* Issue 24, 5 Dec 2001.

2. American Academy of Orthopaedic Surgeons: Sign your site: Wrong site surgery. Rosemont, IL, Web site: www.3.aaos.org/wrong/viewscrp.cfm.

3. Prager L: Mishaps rare, but 100% preventable, surgeons group says. *Los Angeles Times,* 18 Nov 1998.

4. American Academy of Orthopaedic Surgeons: *Advisory Statement: Wrong-Site Surgery.* Web site: www.aaos.org/wordhtml/papers/advistmt/wrong.htm.

5. As quoted in Joint Commission: A follow-up review of wrong site surgery. *Sentinel Event Alert* Issue 24, 5 Dec 2001.

6. New York State Department of Health. Web site: www.health.state.ny.us/nysdoh/commish/2001/preop.htm.

7. Meltzer B: Wrong site surgery: Are your patients at risk? *Outpatient Surgery Magazine* 111:26–35, Feb 2002.

8. Chassin MR, Becher EC: The wrong patient. *Ann Intern Med* 136:826–33, Jun 2002.

9. Joint Commission: Lessons learned: Wrong-site surgery. *Sentinel Event Alert* Issue 6, 28 Aug 1998.

10. Joint Commission: Preventing wrong site surgery: Tips for patients to prevent wrong site surgery. Web site: www.jcaho.org/general+public/patient+safety/preventing+wrong+site+surgery.htm.

11. Surgeons urged to sign patients to avoid surgery on the wrong site. *Healthcare Risk Management* 21:29–31, Mar 1999.

12. Mawji Z, et al: First do no harm: Integrating patient safety and quality improvement. *Jt Comm J Qual Improv* 28:373–86, Jul 2002.

13. Midwest Medical Insurance Company (MMIC): *Risk Management Advisory.* Minneapolis, MN: MMIC, 1997.

14. American Academy of Orthopaedic Surgeons: Report of the task force on wrong-site surgery. Web site: www.aaos.org/wordhtml/meded/tasksite.htm.

CHAPTER 4

PROTECTING PATIENTS FROM MEDICATION ERRORS

The United States is witnessing an era of unparalleled and breathtaking advances in the development of new drugs from new sources. Genetically engineered drugs, which account for the most recent flurry of development activity, are capturing not only Wall Street's attention but also the interest of practitioners and patients nationwide. The range of new and old drugs now available on the market is staggering, well exceeding 10,000 registered products; more than 1,000 new prescription drugs have been introduced since 1975.[1] the Food and Drug Administration (FDA) approved 66 new drugs in 2001 alone, 24 of which were new molecular entities with ingredients never before marketed in the United States.[2]

A critically important component of modern medicine, drugs have made it possible to treat and indeed cure many previously intractable diseases. This has contributed to the increased life expectancy experienced in the United States and elsewhere and has fueled an unprecedented growth in the number of prescriptions dispensed to an increasingly expectant patient and provider marketplace. According to recent data, annual retail pharmaceutical sales in North America reached $147 billion in 2002, up 15% from the previous year; the world market experienced sales of $264 billion.[3] More than three billion prescriptions were dispensed in U.S. community pharmacies in 2001.[4] "With such volume, even small error rates have large potential consequences—an error rate of 1% endangers several million patients," notes one author.[5]

The use of prescription drugs has indeed skyrocketed. Many if not most people who take prescription drugs take multiple medications. Data on the use of prescription drugs in long term care settings indicate that, on average, residents take eight prescription drugs per day.[6] In ambulatory care settings, an estimated two-thirds of office visits end with prescriptions.[7] A study conducted in medical practices in the Boston area indicated that 79% of individuals surveyed reported prescription drug use.[8] Indeed, most encounters between physicians and patients involve medications of some sort. As the baby-boom population ages, the use of prescription medications is expected to continue its upward trend.

Because of their prevalence in medical care and their demonstrated potential for unintended consequences, drugs demand and deserve a high level of attention. With the growth in the development and production of new drugs and dosage forms, health professionals find it challenging to keep abreast of the latest advances. The growth in over-the-counter medications and herbal medicines also make it challenging for health care professionals to keep abreast of adverse drug–drug and drug–food interactions. Recent demographic trends and the fact that the elderly constitute the fastest-growing segment of the nation's population have contributed to skyrocketing medication use rates. Because of the wide range of chemical drug compounds and the variety of human responses to drugs intended to diagnose, prevent, or treat disease, medications are inherently risky. Given the explosion in medication use, is it any wonder that medication errors occur?

Cause for Concern

Medication errors occur with alarming frequency. Although such errors infrequently result in death or serious injury, those that do shake the foundation of public confidence in health care and increase health care costs. In fact, the results of a recent national survey indicate that worries about medication-related issues, such as drug interactions and medication errors, dominate Americans' concerns about visits to health care organizations.[9] Of the top five concerns expressed by individuals, being given two or more medicines that interact in a negative way ranks first (70%), being given the wrong medicine ranks second (69%), and experiencing harmful side effects from taking a medication ranks fifth (67%). A public opinion survey conducted for the NPSF found that medication errors ranked second in types of mistakes experienced by respondents, with 28% of respondents indicating that they had experienced medication errors in health care settings.[10]

A *medication error* is defined by the National Coordinating Council for Medication Error Reporting and Prevention (NCC MERP), an independent body that comprises 19 national organizations, including JCAHO, as

> Any preventable event that may cause or lead to inappropriate medication use or patient harm while the medication is in the control of the health care professional, patient, or consumer. Such events may be related to professional practice, health care products, procedures, and systems, including prescribing; order communication; product labeling, packaging, and nomenclature; compounding; dispensing; distribution; administration; education; monitoring; and use.[11]

The health care literature is full of other closely related terms that warrant definition as well, including *adverse drug event* (ADE), *adverse drug reaction* (ADR), and *medication misadventure*. An ADE is an injury resulting from a medication or lack of an intended medication.[12,13] An ADR is

any unexpected, unintended, undesired, or excessive response to a drug, with or without an injury.[13] An ADR negatively affects prognosis and may result in temporary or permanent harm, disability, or death. It may or may not be the result of a medication error, such as with a medication side effect. Response to an ADR may require a range of actions, including admitting an individual to a health care facility, providing supportive treatments, discontinuing the medicine, changing the medication therapy, or modifying the dose.

This chapter focuses on strategies physicians can use to prevent medication errors that, through omission or commission, lead to or could lead to patient harm.

Medication errors are frequently categorized and studied according to when they occur in the medication use system (see Sidebar 4-1, page 69). For example, one study found that 39% of serious medication errors occurred in the prescribing process, 50% in the order transcription and drug administration processes, and 11% during the dispensing process.[14] Errors frequently involve multiple stages of the drug use process. This is primarily because the medication use function involves many different types of health care professionals, each interacting at different points in the medication use process.

Data from the Joint Commission's sentinel event database, including more than 1,600 sentinel events reviewed by the organization from January 1995 through May 2002, indicate that medication errors accounted for 11.5% of sentinel events.[15] Only suicide (17.1%) and operative/postoperative errors and complications (12.2%) surpassed medication errors as a proportion of the total. As of May 2002, 190 medication errors had been reviewed by JCAHO. The Joint Commission considers any use of medication to restrain an individual to be an inappropriate use of medications.

The Physician's Role

The physician's role in the medication use process is a central one. Physicians and other health care prescribers assess the individual receiving care to determine the appropriate drug therapy. They then select the appropriate drug(s) and therapeutic regimen, checking for potential medication interactions and adverse reactions. They discuss the medication(s) selected and then order the drug(s), communicating medication choices to appropriate staff in their own offices, hospitals or other health care organizations, and pharmacies. Finally, they monitor the individual's clinical condition to determine the effect of the drug(s), and they reevaluate the drug selection, regimen, frequency, and duration, as necessary.

The physician's role is not a simple one. Consider the perspective offered by one author:

> The first-year medical student faces a Herculean task; memorizing all of the important facts about every drug class while learning about anatomy, biochemistry, genetics, and microbiology. The problem is compounded when the young physician begins seeing patients. Now each drug has one or several brand names in addition to the generic name learned during the first year. Drug doses must be modified depending on the patient's size, age, health, or other medications. The practicing physician adapts to this complexity. He or she becomes intimately familiar with all of the drugs in his or her specialty—for example, the cardiologist can explain the subtle differences between each of the dozen calcium-channel blockers. But the same cardiologist rarely treats bladder infections, so she focuses on only one antibiotic to use routinely while forgetting the details of the alternatives. The practicing primary care physician, however, doesn't have the luxury of narrowing his knowledge to a few diseases, so he adapts by focusing on a single medication for each disease. That strategy often fails, because to comply with multiple managed care and hospital formularies, physicians must write prescriptions for less familiar "preferred" medicines.[5]

Sidebar 4-1. The Medication Use System

An expert panel convened by the Joint Commission defined the *medication use system* as, "the safe, effective, appropriate, and efficient use of medications." It commences with *drug selecting and procuring* by an interdisciplinary team, including clinicians and administrators, and advances through *drug prescribing* by the practitioner; *drug preparation and dispensing* by the pharmacist; *drug administering* by the nursing and other health professional staff; and *drug therapy monitoring* by the nursing, medical, and pharmacy staffs.

One or more of these stages occur in most organizations providing health care services. The five processes share the common goal of safe, effective, appropriate, and efficient provision of drug therapy to individuals receiving care. The objective is to provide the "six rights"— the *right* dose of the *right* drug to the *right* individual via, or by, the *right* route at the *right* time with the *right* results.

Source: Nadzam DM: A systems approach to medication use. In Cousins DD (ed): *Medication Use: A Systems Approach to Reducing Errors.* Oakbrook Terrace, IL: Joint Commission on Accreditation of Healthcare Organizations, 1998, p 7.

The role played by physicians is exceedingly complex and highly interrelated with the roles played by administrators, pharmacists, and nurses.

Common Systems Failures

The causes of medication errors cross disciplinary boundaries and reflect system failures, as outlined in Table 4-1, page 71. The Joint Commission's sentinel event database provides one categorization for root cause, systems-oriented error sources. Among the most frequently identified categories are the following:
- Orientation/training,
- Communication,
- Information availability,

- Standardization,
- Storage/access,
- Competency/credentialing,
- Supervision,
- Staffing levels,
- Labeling, and
- Distraction.

A chart illustrating the percentage of medication errors reported to the Joint Commission since January 1995 attributed to each system failure appears as Figure 4-1, page 72. Note that for most medication errors, multiple root causes were identified.

Other categorizations are helpful as well. The major cause and contributing factors categories outlined in *The NCC MERP Taxonomy of Medication Errors* reported to MedMARx, the U.S. Pharmacopeia's Internet-accessible database, include performance deficit; procedure/protocol not followed; knowledge deficit; documentation inaccurate/lacking; communication confusing/intimidating/lacking; transcription inaccurate/omitted; computer entry, drug distribution system, and system safeguards inadequate/lacking; and handwriting illegible/unclear.

A thorough look at important systems-related root causes, as identified by the Joint Commission, and the roles and responsibilities of physicians as team members are critical to both developing a systems approach to error prevention and targeting improvement opportunities. The remaining sections in this chapter focus on the role the physician plays in preventing medication errors and implementing proactive safety strategies to reduce the risk of harm to patients.

System Solution 1: Communication

Sentinel Event Example: Poor Communication

A 60-year-old man receiving home care services complains about a headache to his home health nurse on each of the nurse's three visits during a one-week period. The man indicates that he is tired of "bothering" his primary care physician about various symptoms. At the conclusion of the third visit, the nurse offers to discuss the man's complaint with his primary care physician upon return to the agency. When the nurse discusses the headache with the man's physician, the physician instructs the nurse to call the local pharmacy with the following prescription:

> *Fioricet Tabs. #30*
> *Sig: 1–2 tabs q 4–6 hours prn headache*
> *Refill x3*

In error, the nurse telephones the pharmacy and provides the following prescription:

> *Fiorinal Tabs. #30*
> *Sig: 1–2 tabs q 4–6 hours prn headache*
> *Refill x3*

The man has a long history of peptic ulcer disease, which has resulted in several hospitalizations for gastrointestinal bleeding. The man begins taking the Fiorinal, which contains 325 mg aspirin per tablet. The intended medication—Fioricet—in contrast, contains 325 mg acetaminophen per tablet.

The man completes the entire first prescription and 15 tablets of the first refill. At that point, he presents to the emergency room with acute abdominal pain, blood in the stool, and a hemoglobin of 4.9. He is immediately admitted to the ICU. Within hours, he needs life support. After several units of blood and a four-week hospital stay, the man recovers and is able to return to his home.

Effective communication among all health care professionals is critical to an individual's care. Illegible physician handwriting, oral orders that are transcribed or communicated incorrectly, and order transcription account for a large percentage of drug administration errors. Fifteen percent of the medication errors reported to the NCC MERP in one recent year involved illegible handwriting, problems with leading and trailing zeros, misinterpreted abbreviations, and incomplete

Table 4-1. Major Medication Error Causes and Contributing Factors

Causes (first and second level categories only)

Communication
Verbal miscommunication
Written miscommunication
Misinterpretation of the order

Name confusion
Proprietary (trade) name confusion
Established (generic) name confusion

Labeling
Immediate container labels of product—manufacturer, distributor or repackager
Labels of dispensed product—practitioner
Carton labeling of product—manufacturer, distributor or repackager
Package insert
Electronic reference material
Printed reference material
Advertising

Human factors
Knowledge deficit
Performance deficit
Miscalculation of dosage or infusion rate
Computer error
Error in stocking/restocking/cart filling
Drug preparation error
Transcription error

Stress
Fatigue/lack of sleep
Confrontational or intimidating behavior

Packaging/design
Inappropriate packaging or design
Dosage form (tablet/capsule) confusion
Devices

Contributing factors: systems related (first level categories only)
Lighting
Noise level
Frequent interruptions and distractions
Training
Staffing
Lack of availability of health care professional
Assignment or placement of a health care provider or inexperienced personnel
System for covering patient care (for example, floating personnel, agency coverage)
Policies and procedures
Communication systems among health care practitioners
Patient counseling
Floor stock
Pre-printed medication orders
Other

Source: NCC MERP: *The NCC MERP Taxonomy of Medication Errors*, 1998. Reprinted with permission of the National Coordinating Council for Medication Error Reporting and Prevention, © 2002.

medication orders.[16] One health care organization's multidisciplinary team, including pharmacists, nurses, and physicians, recently studied the percentage of oral orders provided by physicians. The team learned that more than 20% of orders during a specified time period were received orally.[17]

Direct communication among the physician prescribing the medication, the pharmacist filling the medication, and the nurse administering the medication is rare. Because oral telephone orders are often a necessity, particularly in alternate care locations, the potential for medication errors due to miscommunication or misinterpretation is high. The shift of health care services to outpatient locations and the home setting increases the likelihood of this type of error. The opportunity for miscommunication between the individual giving the order and the

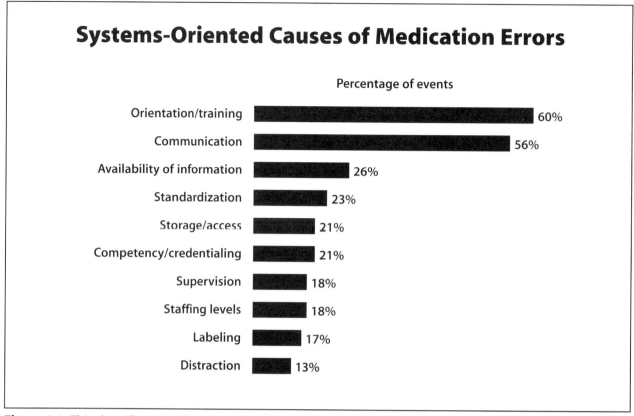

Figure 4-1. This chart illustrates the percentage of medication errors attributed to each system-related root cause, as reviewed by the Joint Commission since January 1995.

clinician receiving the same order is apparent and has resulted in numerous sentinel events throughout the health care field. "[Hand-written prescriptions by prescribers constitute] an uncontrolled process, vulnerable to confusion in interpretation due to unclear writing, misspelling, and lack of consistency and clarity in the writing of drug doses. The process is also confounded by drug trade names which appear similar when hand-written, or sound similar when spoken," notes one team of authors.[18]

Experts nationwide recommend that prescribers move to a direct, computerized order entry system to reduce errors associated with illegible handwriting and look-alike drug names. This strategy is described on page 80.

Prevention Strategy ***Provide clear and complete orders.*** Physicians must ensure that their handwriting is legible and that each medication order is complete. Given the huge number of drugs available on the market, the

opportunity for failure in written communication is enormous. Look-alike names, such as Fiorinal/Fioricet and Cerebyx/Celebrex, are prevalent. Pharmacists and nurses are often left to decipher illegible handwriting and to complete incomplete orders.

Physicians are encouraged to use neat block letters, rather than cursive, and to write each order slowly and carefully.

According to the NCC MERP, complete prescription orders include
- drug name (both brand and generic names);
- exact metric weight or concentration;
- dosage form;
- age and, when appropriate, weight of the patient;
- a brief notation of purpose (for example, for cough), unless considered inappropriate for purposes of maintaining confidentiality; and
- specific directions for use.[19]

Notation of purpose, patient, and weight information create extra safety checks in the medication prescribing and dispensing process. These inexpensive and efficient methods to minimize errors help the pharmacist screen the medication order for proper dose, duration, and appropriateness and may also enable the pharmacist to intervene when multiple prescribers unknowingly order duplicative therapy for the same patient. Listing both the generic and brand names of the drugs on the medication orders provides patients and staff with information to avoid unintentional duplication.[20] For a busy physician who may be seeing 30 to 40 patients per day, these methods, although ideal, may present a significant challenge.

All prescription orders should be written in the metric system, described further in the section on standardization on pages 81 through 83.

 Fax or e-mail orders, to the extent feasible. In such settings as long term care facilities, sending legible orders via facsimile machine can help reduce the likelihood of error and get the prescription into the nurse's hands more quickly. Some organizations use e-mail to transmit physician orders, which requires that the order be typed. Illegible handwriting is not an issue. When orders are sent via fax or e-mail, the staff should be cautioned to take extra care that the information is kept confidential.

 Limit verbal orders. Confusion over the similarity of drug names accounts for approximately 25% of all reports to the USP Medication Errors Reporting (MER) Program.[21] The NCC MERP recommends limiting verbal communication of prescription or medication orders to urgent situations in which immediate written or electronic communication is not feasible.[21]

In a *Sentinel Event Alert* titled "Look-alike, sound-alike drug names," the Joint Commission recommends that health care organizations develop

a policy for taking verbal or telephone orders. For example, when providing a verbal order, one should clearly and slowly state and spell the name of the drug and the dosage ordered. The individual receiving the physician's orders is more likely to misinterpret the order if he or she is not familiar with the drug name and usual dosages. Hence, practitioners should try to limit verbal orders to formulary drugs.

Verbal orders for antineoplastic agents should be avoided at all times due to their complexity and potential to cause sentinel events.

Sidebar 4-2, page 74, outlines the elements that should be included in a verbal order and strategies to ensure error-free communication.

 Request repetition by staff of verbal orders and instructions. Physicians should ask that the full verbal order be read back to them. Although this takes time, it is critical to the accurate transmittal of prescription orders and, hence, to patient safety. Staff working for physicians should be instructed to request and obtain repetition of all verbal orders by the individual receiving the order. This strategy is one of the 2003 National Patient Safety Goals and Recommendations effective for all accreditation programs in January 2003. The full specific recommendation reads, "Implement a process for taking verbal or telephone orders that requires a verification 'read-back' of the complete order by the person receiving the order."[22]

Clarify orders. Be receptive to and available for questions, as feasible. Physicians can encourage all members of the health care team to feel comfortable in questioning them regarding choice of medications, administration routes, dosages, interactions, and reactions. The questioning process serves as an invaluable double-check at the early stages of the medication use process. Order clarification is particularly critical in settings where pharmacists do

Sidebar 4-2. Elements of a Verbal Order and Communication Strategies

- Name of patient
- Age and weight of patient, when appropriate
- Drug name
- Dosage form (for example, tablets, capsules, inhalants)
- Exact strength or concentration
- Dose, frequency, and route
- Quantity and/or duration
- Purpose or indication (unless disclosure is considered inappropriate by the prescriber)
- Specific instructions for use
- Name of prescriber, and telephone number when appropriate
- Name of individual transmitting the order, if different from the prescriber

The content of verbal orders should be clearly communicated. The name of the drug should be confirmed by any of the following:
- Spelling
- Providing both the brand and generic names of the medication
- Providing the indication for use

In order to avoid confusion with spoken numbers, a dose such as 50 mg should be dictated as "fifty milligrams… five zero milligrams" to distinguish from "fifteen milligrams… one five milligrams."

Instructions for use should be provided without abbreviations. For example, "1 tab tid" should be communicated as "Take/give one tablet three times daily."

Source: National Coordinating Council for Medication Error Reporting and Prevention: Recommendations to reduce medication errors associated with verbal medication orders and prescriptions (adopted 20 Feb 2001). © 1998–2002 National Coordinating Council for Medication Error Reporting and Prevention. All rights reserved.

not have an opportunity to review physician orders. For example, nurses in long term care, behavioral health care, and home care organizations frequently communicate physician orders over the telephone to pharmacists in different locations. Physicians should encourage order clarification and make themselves available, as feasible.

 Take extra precaution with error-prone medications through increased communication. The professional literature is full of reports of medications known to have frequently been involved with serious medication errors. According to the ISMP, the five high-alert medications are insulin, opiates and narcotics, injectable potassium chloride (or phosphate) concentrate, intravenous anticoagulants (such as heparin), and sodium chloride solutions above 0.9%.[23] For example, use of trailing zeros with insulin leads to inappropriate administration. An order for Humulin Insulin NPH, written as "10.0 Units SQ AM and PM," can very easily be misinterpreted by the pharmacist and nurse as "100 Units SQ AM and PM." Therefore, physicians and other prescribers should never write insulin orders with trailing zeros (see discussion of standardization pp. 81–83). When there is a trailing zero, the nurse must clarify the order prior to administration. This extra communication is critical. Other risk factors associated with high-alert medications and error reduction strategies that physicians can either implement or for which they can participate in systemwide implementation appear as Table 4-2, page 75.

 Communicate with and educate the individual receiving the medication. A physician should identify for the patient and family, as appropriate, each medication he or she is prescribing. If a new medication is being given, the physician should take time to educate the individual and family about the medication and provide available literature describing the drug (with mention of both its brand and generic names) and side effects that may be experienced. The physician

Table 4-2. High-Alert Medication Safety: Risk Factors and Suggested Error-Reduction Strategies

Insulin

Common risk factors

- Lack of dose check systems
- Insulin and heparin vials kept in close proximity to each other on a nursing unit, leading to mix-ups
- Use of "u" as an abbreviation for "units" in orders (which can be confused with "o," resulting in a 10-fold overdose)
- Incorrect rates being programmed into an infusion pump

Suggested strategies

- Establish a check system whereby one nurse prepares the dose and another nurse reviews it.
- Do not store insulin and heparin near each other.
- Build in an independent check system for infusion pump rates and concentration settings.

Opiates and narcotics

Common risk factors

- Parenteral narcotics stored in nursing areas as floor stock
- Confusion between hydromorphone and morphine
- Patient-controlled analgesia (PCA) errors regarding concentration and rate

Suggested strategies

- Limit the opiates and narcotics available in floor stock.
- Educate staff about hydromorphone and morphine mix-ups.
- Implement PCA protocols that include double-checks of the drug, pump setting, and dosage.

Injectable potassium chloride or phosphate concentrate

Common risk factors

- Storing concentrated potassium chloride/phosphate outside of the pharmacy

- Mixing potassium chloride/phosphate extemporaneously
- Requests for unusual concentrations

Suggested strategies

- Remove potassium chloride/phosphate from floor stock.
- Move drug preparation off units and use commercially available premixed IV solutions.
- Standardize and limit drug concentrations.

Intravenous anticoagulants (heparin)

Common risk factors

- Unclear labeling regarding concentration and total volume
- Multi-dose containers
- Confusion between heparin and insulin due to similar measurement units and proximity

Suggested strategies

- Standardize concentrations and use premixed solutions.
- Use only single-dose containers.
- Separate heparin and insulin and remove heparin from the top of medication carts.

Sodium chloride solutions above 0.9 percent

Common risk factors

- Storing sodium chloride solutions (above 0.9 percent) on nursing units
- Large number of concentrations/formulations available
- No double-check system in place

Suggested strategies

- Limit access of sodium chloride solutions (above 0.9 percent) and remove from nursing units.
- Standardize and limit drug concentrations.
- Double check pump rate, drug, concentration and line attachments.

Source: Joint Commission: High-alert medications and patient safety. *Sentinel Event Alert,* Issue 11, Nov 1999.

should help ensure the patient's and family's understanding by asking them to repeat how and when to take the medication, possible side effects, and what to do if adverse effects occur.

Communication and education in any care setting help to reduce the likelihood that at a later date an individual will receive the incorrect medication or a medication intended for another person or that a dose will be omitted. In addition, individuals with adequate information about medications to which they are allergic will be better able to help prevent future allergic reactions.

Patients undoubtedly are better educated now than ever before regarding medications that may be available to treat their conditions. Direct-to-consumer television, radio, and print advertisements by pharmaceutical companies are playing a considerable part in the education process, as is information available on the Internet. Some experts in the health care industry worry that ads may be inappropriately increasing demand for some new prescription medicines that are costlier than older medicines that work just as well. Patient safety may also be an issue, as patients may request new drugs for unapproved purposes. For these reasons, many physician organizations and specialty societies have gone on record as opposing direct-to-consumer advertising. Physicians should be aware of information that is widely available to consumers and counsel patients on safety-related issues.

Medication compliance is often a critical issue. Physicians can stress as part of the education process the importance of the individual's responsibility regarding medication use. An individual receiving care must be an active partner in the medication use process. He or she must tell the physician about all medicines taken, including over-the-counter medicines such as aspirin, ibuprofen, vitamins, and herbals, as well as any drug allergies.[24]

Physicians can encourage patients to ask questions and express concerns. In its Speak Up campaign,

JCAHO urges physicians and nurses to wear buttons bearing this slogan.

System Solution 2: Collaboration

Example: Pharmacist/Physician Teamwork

A physician wrote an order for Clindamycin oral and Rifampin oral for a child with a staphylococcal infection that is resistant to methicillin. The pharmacist, knowing that Clindamycin oral has the propensity to cause pseudomembraneous colitis in 1 in 30,000 cases and that Rifampin is not normally used to treat a staph infection but to treat tuberculosis, called the physician to clarify the order. The physician indicated that she was using Rifampin as a "potentiator" of Clindamycin to treat staphylococcus aureus resistant to methicillin. The interaction of the two drugs results in a pharmacologic response greater than the sum of individual responses to each drug, so, in effect, Rifampin boosts Clindamycin's therapeutic strength. Furthermore, the physician indicated that pseudomembraneous colitis, although proved to occur in 1 in 30,000 cases due to Clindamycin, was the lesser of side effects from the alternative—intravenous Vancomycin.

Although the importance of team collaboration is described generally in Chapter 1, the concept deserves special focus as a systems solution for reducing medication errors. As integral members of the medication use process team, physicians play a central role in systemwide collaborative solutions. Deborah M. Nadzam, PhD, RN, administrative director of the Quality Institute at the Cleveland Clinic Health System and a key contact for the NCC MERP, describes traditional medication use team members as follows[25]:

• *Administrators and clinicians* are at the "front end" of the process, making decisions regarding the selection, procurement, and storage of drugs according to care and organization needs. They establish formularies, direct the development and implementation of staff education programs, and identify and procure necessary equipment, among other functions.

- *Physicians and other health care prescribers* perform the role described earlier; that is, they assess the individual receiving care to determine the appropriate drug therapy, *select* the appropriate drug(s) and therapeutic regimen, *discuss* medications selected with the patient and family, order the drug(s), *communicate* medication choices to appropriate staff in their own offices, hospitals, or other health care organizations, and pharmacies, *monitor* the individual's clinical condition to determine the effect of the drug, and *reevaluate* the drug selection, regimen, frequency, and duration, as necessary.
- *Pharmacists* procure, store, prepare, and dispense medications and provide information to other professionals regarding established and new drug therapies. They ensure correct labeling and timely and accurate dispensing. In their role as reviewers of all drug orders and prescriptions, they question unusual dosages, routes of administration, and frequencies.
- *Nurses*—who can be many different types of professionals, including licensed practical nurses, registered nurses, clinical nurse specialists, and nurse practitioners—administer medications and are in frequent contact with the individual receiving care. Thus, they are able to note negative side effects.

Individuals receiving care, the recipients of medications, and families or significant others should participate in medication administration and monitoring activities. As described earlier, in the Internet age, familiarity with medications is increasing as stays in health care settings shorten and more care is provided at home. Health care professionals must make the individuals receiving care and their caregivers partners in the medication use process. All team members play a significant role in reducing the likelihood of medication errors.

To achieve optimal patient outcomes related to the delivery of pharmaceutical care, the unique knowledge and competencies of each profession involved in the medication use process must be heard and respected.

 Collaborate with pharmacists. "The purpose of the traditional collaboration between physician and pharmacist in the delivery of pharmaceutical care is to combine the unique knowledge and competencies of each to achieve optimal outcomes in, and for, the patient," writes one team of experts.[26] A collegial, respectful relationship between the physician and the pharmacist in the example on page 76 allowed each to discuss the case intelligently. No intermediaries were used, which facilitated confidentiality between both parties.

Physicians should promote the collaborative role of pharmacists in the prescribing stage. For example, if the pharmacist believes an order is specified for the incorrect dosage or the patient could experience adverse drug interactions, the pharmacist raises the matter with the physician and participates in the issue's resolution. In an ideal world, the physician collaborates with the pharmacist to develop, implement, and monitor a therapeutic plan to produce defined therapeutic outcomes for the patient.[27] In the role of therapeutic consultant, the pharmacist can participate in and positively influence decisions related to selecting the right drug, dosage, frequency, and route of drug therapy. This role affords the prescriber the opportunity to obtain information on new drugs from the pharmacist. Pharmacokinetic consultations provided to physicians on certain drugs, such as Vancomycin, aminoglycosides, aminophylline, digoxin, clozapine, phenytoin, and warfarin, are common and critical to the prevention of medication errors.

The usefulness of drug therapy recommendations from clinical pharmacists is well documented in the professional literature. One study indicated that family practice physicians in a family medicine clinic rated 88% of pharmacist recommendations as "very useful."[28] The recommendations called for as many as three actions to be taken by a physician. Again, 88% of patients were rated by physicians as improved clinically because of the recommendations.

Physicians and nurses have been making rounds together for years. Pharmacist participation on rounds can make a positive contribution to the prevention of medication selection and prescribing errors. The pharmacist's participation in drug therapy decisions during rounds at the time of prescribing has been documented in the professional literature to prevent medication errors and reduce drug use, resulting in improved care and reduced costs.[29–31] The 1999 study by Leape and colleagues noted significant medication error reduction (66%) achieved by pharmacist participation on an ICU patient care team. Physicians accepted nearly all (99%) of the pharmacist recommendations tracked in the study.[29]

In the ambulatory clinic setting, physicians interact closely and successfully with pharmacists through specialized pharmacist-staffed clinics, such as diabetes management clinics, anticoagulation clinics, or compliance clinics.[32] Physicians "refer" patients to the pharmacist in such clinics to receive further follow-up assessment, medication use review, and medication monitoring. Such clinics foster collegial interaction between physicians and pharmacists and allow more efficient use of both practitioners' time.

Physician–pharmacist collaboration is gaining needed ground. A newly released report of the Medicare Payment Advisory Commission recommended that the Department of Health and Human Services assess models of physician–pharmacist collaboration to manage the medication needs of Medicare beneficiaries.[33]

Prevention Strategy *Collaborate with nurses.* Physician–nurse collaboration is crucial to patient safety at all stages of the medication use process. At the prescribing stage, nurses ask questions and clarify any unclear orders. Nurses serve as the final check to ensure that the pharmacy has delivered what the prescriber ordered and that the order appears appropriate, given the individual's condition, allergies, and other factors. They assess the individual receiving care to determine whether a change in condition warrants withholding the medication. They serve as frontline advocates for care recipients, communicating and coordinating with other health care professionals to help ensure that required adjustments to care plans and care provision are made.

As frontline advocates for the individuals they serve, nurses are, in fact, the "sentinels" of care, sounding the warning to physicians and other health care team members for those in need of help and providing the help, as needed and feasible. On individual and leadership bases, physicians should do their part to ensure full recognition of the important patient safety role played by nurses and the critical nature of physician–nurse collaboration. They can also play an important part in helping to identify nurse staffing shortages that could affect patient safety.

System Solution 3: Technology and Information Management

As mentioned in Chapter 1, when designed and used properly, technology can aid a physician's quest for improved patient safety. Computers are capable of managing reams of information and making it available at the point of care. "The problem that many hospitals and physicians face now is that there are huge amounts of information available. That much material can be negative in the sense that people just don't know where to start," says one writer.[34] The result is often that they do not start the process of developing and implementing computer-based information systems. The lack of critical information, in fact, was cited as a root cause of 26% of sentinel events reviewed by the Joint Commission.

CPOE, or electronic prescribing, is one use of technology that has proven effective in reducing medication errors associated with prescribing. As described in Chapter 1, most patient safety–related organizations are calling for its use by physicians and for its implementation across all types of health care organizations.

The reality, however, is that virtually all prescriptions in the United States are still handwritten.[35] All though CPOE systems are being introduced into health care, it is estimated that currently fewer than 5% of U.S. physicians use these systems to write their prescriptions electronically.[36] Even in hospitals, the rate of electronic prescribing is low. A study of CPOE use within hospitals in one southern state indicated rates as low as 21.9%.[37] Barriers to increased use are formidable. Indeed, capabilities of online prescription technologies are outpacing acceptance. Cost of developing and maintaining computer systems is a significant barrier, as is acceptance of new, "nontraditional" methods. Most physicians' offices are computerized, but only for billing and practice management functions and not for clinical functions. The link between prescriber offices and pharmacies is in early developmental stages. Most pharmacies are computerized but have not developed the ability to receive electronic prescriptions because of lack of computerization on the prescriber end.[38] To better ensure a fail-safe prescription ordering system, all pharmacies should be equipped with computer capabilities to accept physician orders. Some suggest involving adjudication of medication orders by third-party insurers. After the patient selects a pharmacy, the insurer would send authorized prescriptions to the pharmacy electronically.

"One expert speculates that online prescribing will be the killer app [pivotal application] of the electronic medical record—a particular application that has such inherent value that it gets people moving. He thinks that, just as word processing was the application that brought computers to nearly every desktop, online prescribing may be the driving force behind computerizing clinical practice," notes

---

Sidebar 4-3. Barriers to Use of Computerized Physician Order Entry

The American Society of Health-System Pharmacists cites the following barriers to increased use of computerized medication-order entry:
- Cost.
- Reluctance of prescribers to give up long established and comfortable manual processes for prescribing.
- Inconsistencies in system availability in different arenas of practice. For example, prescribers would be more likely to use computerized medication-order-entry systems if they were standardized across all sites of practice.
- A lack of voice-activated computer technology for medication-order entry.
- A tendency for hospitals to apply computerization first to business affairs rather than clinical service support.
- Prescribers' lack of computer skills.
- Design weaknesses in computer systems.

Source: Top-priority actions for preventing adverse drug events in hospitals: Recommendations of an expert panel. *Am J Health-Syst Pharm* 53:747–51, 1 Apr 1996. American Society of Health-System Pharmacists, Inc., All rights reserved. Reprinted with permission (R0244).

---

one author.[38] Barriers to CPOE cited by the American Society of Health-System Pharmacists (ASHP) appear as Sidebar 4-3, above. As mentioned earlier, online prescribing is not the panacea for medication errors at the prescribing stage. Errors can occur even with online prescribing.

 Prevention Strategy ***Learn to use electronic prescribing technologies.*** Because it offers the hope for significantly reduced medication errors on a consistent basis, use of electronic prescribing systems by physicians is needed in both inpatient and outpatient settings. Two experts describe the future use of such systems in ambulatory environments:

Prescribing technologies should have a managed care organization's medication formulary entered in the system. As the prescriber enters that patient's name on his or her computer screen, the appropriate formulary should be in place. Prescribers should no longer be distracted by having to deal with changes in prescription that are brought about by revised formulary decisions. When a non-formulary class medication is prescribed, the computer prescribing program should automatically suggest alternative formulary agents that can be used.[39]

The cost of handheld technology for electronic prescribing in the office setting is falling and, generally, is no longer prohibitively expensive for individual physicians. PDAs are relatively easy for physicians to use. One manufacturer offers a device that checks for allergies and drug interactions, matches the diagnosis and drug therapy, provides managed care formulary information, and allows physicians to send orders to local pharmacies electronically. Physicians can consult their specialty organizations for educational sessions and information on appropriate electronic prescribing technologies.

Physicians can learn much by reviewing the experience of organizations that have implemented CPOE. For example, Brigham and Women's Hospital implemented CPOE nearly ten years ago. Alerts and reminder features built into the system include duplicate checking, drug–allergy interaction checking, drug–drug interaction checking, and guidelines regarding medications, dosing restrictions for potassium chloride, renal dosing, and chemotherapy. "The change from paper-based ordering to computerized ordering generated some angst among physicians, nurses, and pharmacists, but the providers adapted within a few weeks," comments one expert team.[40] The cost for the system was $1.4 million, but the organization expects to save at least $5 million annually by raising the caliber of care.[41]

 Help ensure the proper interface of CPOE systems. Physicians and the organization in which they work need to exercise caution in ensuring that the CPOE systems they select and implement properly interface with the pharmacy's computerized systems. Some standalone CPOE systems available in the marketplace allow physicians to enter data while on the unit, in their offices, and so forth but do not directly interface with the organization's pharmacy system. This means that, although the physician order is neatly transcribed by the computer, the physician is not able to receive information such as allergy warnings, drug interaction warnings, or dose range checking that is available through the pharmacy computerized system. Such standalone CPOE systems may give nurses, administrators, and other health care team members a false sense of security, which could lead to the administration of initial medication doses before pharmacy review. Orders must always go through the pharmacy system's normal review process.

 Consider using computer-aided medication selection systems. Paired with the clinical knowledge of the prescribing physician, computer-aided medication selection can help prevent adverse events, promote optimal care decisions, and reduce costs. CDSSs display drug use guidelines, offer relevant alternatives, and suggest appropriate doses and frequencies (see Chapter 1, page 28).

 Ensure capture and availability of critical medication-related information. The availability of needed information related to medications is critical to patient safety. "Physicians need to become involved in improving the quality of all the systems used in their practices—not just the refill system, but the prescribing system and the laboratory and radiology follow-up systems," suggests physician-researcher David Bates.[42] All physicians must ensure access to reliable and current drug information. Sidebar 4-4, page 81, provides the "low-tech" tips for reducing medication-related adverse events offered to physicians by the staff of RMF of the Harvard Medical Institutions.

System Solution 4: Standardization

Sentinel Event Example: Medication Error

An 85-year-old woman is admitted to the hospital because she has blood in her stool. Her physician schedules a colonoscopy for the following morning and writes a prescription for Ativan (lorazepam) 1.0 mg to be administered 30 minutes prior to the procedure. During the past year, the hospital's nursing staff noted that lorazepam had been missing from several unit-dose drawers. Hence, the medication is now issued on a count sheet for general unit use and, because it is a controlled substance, is documented as a CII narcotic.

The nurse interprets the care recipient's dose as 10 mg rather than 1.0 mg because the physician had placed a terminal zero after a decimal point. Because the physician ordered the medication to be given as soon as possible, and because the medication is maintained in narcotic floor stock, the order is not reviewed by a pharmacist prior to administration. The nurse removes ten 1 mg tablets from the locked area of the medication cart and proceeds to the care recipient's room. The alert elderly lady questions why she is being given so many tablets. The nurse reassures her that preoperative medications are typically given in higher doses than usual.

In addition to lorazepam, the woman is receiving both furosemide and lisinopril for treatment of congestive heart failure. Both medications lower her blood pressure. When the incorrect 10 mg lorazepam dose is added to these routine medications administered less than one hour earlier, the woman suffers a cardiac arrest, and she dies later that afternoon.

One of the major causes of medication errors is the ongoing use of potentially dangerous abbreviations and dose expressions.[43] Underlying factors contributing to many of these errors are clinicians'

Sidebar 4-4. Tips for Improving Office Practice Systems to Reduce Medication-Related Adverse Events

- Maintain a medication record to track all medications, including dosages, prescribed by you and other providers.
- Develop a list of medications that warrant close monitoring.
- Document all sample medications given to patients.
- To prevent or identify drug toxicity, create a tickler file to schedule patient visits at regular intervals for blood tests or diagnostic exams.
- Review the patient's record prior to prescribing renewals. Sign-off on renewals is recommended.
- Update patient drug allergies at every clinical encounter. Known allergies should be conspicuously flagged.
- Be aware of cross-sensitivities for patients who have drug allergies.
- Ask the patient at every clinical encounter if she/he is taking any new medications, including over-the-counter drugs, vitamins, or homeopathics.
- If the patient is being seen in a specialty clinic such as an anticoagulant clinic, establish communication and clarify roles between the primary care physician and the consulting physician.

Source: Tips for improving office practice systems to reduce adverse events. *Forum* 20(2):6–7, Feb 2000. Used with permission of the Risk Management Foundation of the Harvard Medical Institutions.

---

illegible or confusing handwriting and the failure of health care providers to communicate clearly with one another. Standardization of abbreviations and dose expressions is vitally needed to ensure patient safety. Supervising physicians in teaching hospitals need to be particularly attentive to varying or new abbreviations used by house staff and students. Use of these should be discontinued.

Despite repeated warnings for more than 25 years by the ISMP and other organizations about the dangers associated with using certain abbreviations when communicating medication information, the practice of using these dangerous abbreviations continues, increasing the potential for patient harm. "Symbols and abbreviations are frequently used to save time and effort when writing prescriptions and documenting in patient charts," says the JCAHO's associate director of surveyor development and management. "However, some symbols and abbreviations have the potential for misinterpretation or confusion."

Examples of especially problematic abbreviations include *U* for *units* and *μg* for *micrograms*. When *U* is handwritten, it can often look like a zero. There are numerous case reports where the root cause of a sentinel event related to insulin dosage has been the interpretation of a *U* as a zero. Using the abbreviation *μg* instead of *mcg* has also been the source of errors because when handwritten, the symbol *μ* can look like an *m*. The use of trailing zeros (for example, 2.0 versus 2) and of a leading decimal point without a leading zero (for example, .2 instead of 0.2) are other dangerous order-writing practices. The decimal point is sometimes not seen when orders are handwritten using trailing zeros or no leading zeros. Misinterpretation of such orders could lead to ten-fold dosing errors. "To minimize the potential for error and to maximize patient safety, prescribers need to avoid such specifically dangerous abbreviations and phrases," says the associate director.

Following the tragic death of an infant due to the misinterpretation of a prescription for morphine, the ISMP recently issued an alert to health care institutions, reminding them of the dangers of using certain dangerous abbreviations and dose expressions.[44] "ISMP and others have advocated abandoning the use of these abbreviations and expressions for almost three decades," says Michael Cohen, president of the ISMP. "ISMP has also stressed that it is equally important to avoid these dangerous abbreviations and dose expressions in other communications such as

computer-generated labels, Medication Administration Records (MARs), labels for drug storage bins/shelves, preprinted orders and protocols, and pharmacy and prescriber order entry screens."[44]

Sidebar 4-5, page 83, presents the NCC MERP's observations concerning dangerous abbreviations and dose expressions most often associated with misinterpretation and patient harm (as reported to the USP-ISMP MER Program).

The following strategies are recommended by NCC MERP.[45]

 Use the metric system when writing prescription orders. "All prescription orders should be written in the metric system except for therapies that use standard units such as insulin or vitamins. Units should be spelled out rather than writing 'U.' The change to the use of the metric system from the archaic apothecary and avoirdupois systems will help avoid misinterpretations of these abbreviations and symbols, and miscalculations when converting to metric, which is used in product labeling and package inserts," notes NCC MERP.[45]

 Ensure proper use of leading and trailing zeros. "A leading zero should always precede a decimal expression of less than one. A terminal or trailing zero should never be used after a decimal. Ten-fold errors in drug strength and dosage have occurred with decimals due to the use of a trailing zero or the absence of a leading zero," notes the NCC MERP.[45]

 Work with other physicians and organization staff, including pharmacists, to develop a list of abbreviations, acronyms, and symbols used throughout the organization, including a list of abbreviations, acronyms, and symbols not to use . Comply with the agreed-upon no-use policy. This strategy is one of the 2003 National Patient Safety Goals and Recommendations effective for all JCAHO accreditation programs in

---

Sidebar 4-5. NCC MERP Observations Regarding Dangerous Abbreviations

Abbreviation (intended meaning): Common Error

- U (units): Mistaken as a zero or a four (4) resulting in overdose. Also mistaken for "cc" (cubic centimeters) when poorly written.
- µg (Micrograms): Mistaken for "mg" (milligrams) resulting in a ten-fold overdose.
- Q.D. (Latin abbreviation for every day): The period after the "Q" has sometimes been mistaken for a "1," and the drug has been given "QID" (four times daily) rather than daily.
- Q.O.D. (Latin abbreviation for every other day): Misinterpreted as "QD" (daily) or "QID" (four times daily). If the "O" is poorly written, it looks like a period or "1."
- SC or SQ (subcutaneous): Mistaken as "SL" (sublingual) when poorly written.
- T I W (Three times a week): Misinterpreted as "three times a day" or "twice a week."
- D/C (discharge; also discontinue): Patient's medications have been prematurely discontinued when D/C (intended to mean "discharge") was misinterpreted as "discontinue," because it was followed by a list of drugs.
- HS (half strength): Misinterpreted as the Latin abbreviation "HS" (hour of sleep).
- cc (cubic centimeters): Mistaken as "U" (units) when poorly written.
- AU, AS, AD (Latin abbreviation for both ears; left ear; right ear): Misinterpreted as the Latin abbreviation "OU" (both eyes); "OS" (left eye); "OD" (right eye).
- Prescribers should not use vague instructions such as "take as directed" or "take/use as needed" as the sole direction for use. Specific directions to the patient are useful to help reinforce proper medication use, particularly if therapy is to be interrupted for a time. Clear directions are a necessity for the dispenser to (1) check the proper dose for the patient; and (2) enable effective patient counseling.

These abbreviations are particularly dangerous because they have been consistently misunderstood and therefore, should never be used. The Council reviewed the uses for many abbreviations and determined that any attempt at standardization of abbreviations would not adequately address the problems of illegibility and misuse.

July 2002. "Prescribers should avoid use of abbreviations including those for drug names (for example, MOM, HCTZ) and Latin directions for use," notes the NCC MERP.[45]

 Identify and use relevant clinical practice guidelines. As described in Chapter 1, pages 24–27, clinical practice guidelines aim at standardization of practice. When well conceived, they can improve care quality and safety and communication among care providers. Some organizations, for example, have implemented therapeutic guidelines for heparin and warfarin use, certain antibiotics, and insulin for pregnant mothers.[46]

System Solution 5: Education

Errors in prescribing, as noted earlier, account for 39% of serious medication errors. Experts have classified prescribing errors in a number of different ways. Lucian Leape and his colleagues indicate that the most common cause of error is a lack of complete knowledge about drugs. This is followed by the lack of available patient information, and the third most common error is slips or lapses of memory.[14] The latter frequently result from interruptions, rushing, stress, and fatigue. One medication errors expert classifies prescribing errors as having to do with issues of knowledge, concentration, and communication.[47] Communication errors involve problems of order legibility and use of abbreviations and acronyms. One writer notes, "A large number of errors appeared to result from a lack of knowledge or appreciation of drug therapy issues—misapplication of drug therapy rules (such as ordering 40 mEq of potassium chloride intravenous push)—as well as apparent mental lapses and mental slips."[48]

Lack of knowledge is the foremost cause of prescribing errors. "Giving the patient an overdose (41%) or an insufficient dose (17%), missing an allergy warning (13%), giving the wrong dosage form (12%), or duplicating treatment (5%) were the major reasons for prescribing errors [in one study]," notes one expert.[5]

Lesar et al note that "improved education and training of all medical professionals in the use of medications are likely to have a positive impact, primarily by increasing the level of appreciation for applying the information in practice and increasing the chance of error detection."[48]

 Learn, keep up to date, and use the principles of safe prescribing. Medical school graduates may not have received adequate education about general pharmacology and safe prescribing practices.[18] Physicians must supplement their formal education with continuing professional education and reading related to medication usage. Medical staff directors can consider offering medical staff in-services on the latest in safe prescribing practices and other topics.

 Enlist the help of other clinicians in the education process. Physicians can turn to pharmacists to assist their educational objectives related to safe medication prescribing. Pharmacists can help address the knowledge deficit by ensuring that prescribers have timely information about established and new drug therapies, dosage changes, dosage forms, and other such information.

Closing Comments

As key players in the medication use process, physicians can proactively help prevent medication errors. Proper continuing education and credentialing ensure that physicians are knowledgeable about medication prescribing and error reduction techniques. Enhanced communication and collaboration among physicians, nurses, pharmacists, and patients and their families can prevent errors at the prescribing stage of the medication use process. Clear and complete orders are critical to patient safety. Electronic prescribing and standardization are proven techniques to reduce prescribing errors. Physicians can pursue strategies in each area to reduce the likelihood of harm to patients in their care.

REFERENCES

1. Proulx S, Wilfinger R, Cohen MR: Medication error prevention: Profiling one of pharmacy's foremost advocacy efforts for advice on error prevention. *Pharm Pract Manage Q* 17(1):1–9, 1997.

2. U.S. Food and Drug Administration: Improving public health: Promoting safe and effective drug use. Web site: www.fda.gov/opacom/factsheets/justthefacts/3cder.html.

3. IMS Health World Drug Monitor: News release. Jun 2002. Web site: www.imshealth.com/public/structure/dispcontent/1,2779,1000-1000-144238,00.html.

4. National Association of Chain Drug Stores: In 2001 retail pharmacies filled over 3 billion prescriptions totaling $164 billion (news release). 12 Aug 2002. Web site: www.nacds.org/wmspage.cfm?parm1=2489.

5. Newcomer LN: Medicare pharmacy coverage: Ensuring safety before funding. *Health Affairs* 19:59–62, Mar/Apr 2000.

6. American Society of Consultant Pharmacists: *A Model Long-Term Care Pharmacy Benefit,* 1996. Web site: www.ascp.com/member/policy/mltcpb.

7. White MK: Patient adherence. Presented at the Medication Errors Symposium, Baltimore, MD, 7–8 Apr 2000.

8. Gandhi TK, et al: Drug complications in outpatients. *J Gen Intern Med* 15:149–54, Mar 2000.

9. American Society of Health-System Pharmacists: Survey reveals patient concerns about medication-related issues. (press release). 17 Jul 2002. Web site: www.ashp.com/public/news/releases/ShowReleases.cfm?id=2996.

10. National Patient Safety Foundation at the American Medical Association: *Public Opinion of Patient Safety Issues: Research Findings.* Sep 1997. Web site: www.npsf.org/html/presrel/finalrpt.pdf.

11. National Coordinating Council for Medication Error Reporting and Prevention: About medication errors. Web site: www.nccmerp.org/aboutmederrors.htm.

12. Bates DW, et al: Incidence of adverse drug events and potential adverse drug events. *JAMA* 274(1):29–34, 1995.

13. American Society of Health-System Pharmacists: Suggested definitions and relationships among medication misadventures, medication errors, adverse drug events, and adverse drug reactions. Web site: www.ashp.com/public/proad/mederror/draftdefin.html.

14. Leape LL, et al: Systems analysis of adverse drug events. *JAMA* 274:35–43, 5 Jul 1995.

15. Joint Commission statistics provide insight into causes of sentinel events. *Jt Comm Persp* 22:3–5, Aug 2002.

16. National Coordinating Council for Medication Error Reporting and Prevention: Council identifies and makes recommendations to improve error-prone aspects of prescription writing. Rockville, MD: United States Pharmacopeial Convention, 4 Sep 1996. Referenced in Meyer TA: Improving the quality of the order-writing process for inpatient prescriptions. *Am J Health-Syst Pharm* 57(Suppl 4)S18–S22, 15 Dec 2000.

17. Meyer TA: Improving the quality of the order-writing process for inpatient orders and outpatient prescriptions. *Am J Health-Syst Pharm* 57(Suppl 4):S18–S22, 15 Dec 2000.

18. Thornton PD, Simon S, Mathew TH: Towards safer drug prescribing, dispensing and administration in hospitals. *J Qual Clin Practice* 19:41–5, Mar 1999.

19. National Coordinating Council for Medication Error Reporting and Prevention: Recommendations to correct error-prone aspects of prescription writing (adopted 4 Sep 1996). Web site: www.nccmerp.org.

20. Joint Commission: Look-alike, sound-alike drug names. *Sentinel Event Alert* Issue 19, May 2001.

21. National Coordinating Council for Medication Error Reporting and Prevention: Recommendations to reduce medication errors associated with verbal medication orders and prescriptions (adopted 20 Feb 2001). Web site: www.nccmerp.org.

22. Joint Commission: JCAHO approves National Patient Safety Goals for 2003. *Jt Comm Persp* 22:1–3, Sep 2002.

23. Cohen MR, Kilo CM: High-alert medications: Safeguarding against errors. In Cohen MR (ed): *Medication Errors.* Washington, DC: American Pharmaceutical Association, 1999, pp 5.1–5.40.

24. Joint Commission: Five steps to safer health care. Web site: www.jcaho.org/general+public/patient+safety/5+steps.htm.

25. Nadzam DM: A systems approach to medication use. In Cousins DD (ed): *Medication Use: A Systems Approach to Reducing Errors.* Oakbrook Terrace, IL: Joint Commission, 1998.

26. Rupp MT, DeYoung M, Schondelmeyer SW: Prescribing problems and pharmacist interventions in community practice. *Med Care* 30(10):926–40, 1992.

27. Hepler CD, Strand LM: Opportunities and responsibilities in pharmaceutical care. *Am J Hosp Pharm* 47:533–43, Mar 1990.

28. Haxby DG, Weart CW, Goodman BW: Family practice physicians' perceptions of the usefulness of drug therapy recommendations from clinical pharmacists. *Am J Hosp Pharm* 45(4):824–7, 1988.

29. Leape LL, et al: Pharmacist participation on physician rounds and adverse drug events in the intensive care unit. *JAMA* 282(3):267–70, 1999.

30. Montazeri M, Cook DJ: Impact of a clinical pharmacist in a multidisciplinary intensive care unit. *Crit Care Med* 22:1044–8, Jun 1994.

31. Pantaleo N, Talan M: Applying the performance improvement team concept to the medication order process. *J for Healthcare Qual* 20(2):30–5, 1998.

32. Raish DW: Patient counseling in community pharmacy and its relationship with prescription payment methods and practice settings. *Ann Pharmacother* 27(10):1173–9, 1993.

33. American Society of Health-System Pharmacists: Congressional advisory commission recognizes value of pharmacist–physician collaboration. (press release). 27 Jun 2002. Web site: www.ashp.com/public/news/releases.

34. As quoted in Voelker R: Hospital collaborative creates tools to help reduce medication errors. *JAMA* 286:3067–9, 26 Dec 2001.

35. Schiff GD, Rucker TD: Computerized prescribing: Building the electronic infrastructure for better medication usage. *JAMA* 279(13):1024–9, 1998.

36. Joint Commission: Medication errors related to potentially dangerous abbreviations. *Sentinel Event Alert* Issue 23, Sep 2001.

37. Lin B, Anderson LR: The role of the pharmacy department in the prevention of adverse drug events: A survey of current practices. *Pharm Pract Manage Q* 17(1):10–6, 1997.

38. Binius T: Ability to prescribe on-line growing faster than acceptance. *Am Medical News,* 20 April 1998.

39. Armstrong EP, Chrischilles EA: Electronic prescribing and monitoring are needed to improve drug use. *Arch Int Med* 160:2713–4, 9 Oct 2000.

40. Kuperman GJ, et al: Patient safety and computerized medication ordering at Brigham and Women's Hospital. *J Qual Improve* 27:509–21, Oct 2001.

41. Haugh R: To the rescue. *Hosp Health Network* pp 44–8, Apr 2000.

42. Bates DW: A 40-year old woman who noticed a medication error. *JAMA* 285:3134–40, 27 Jun 2001.

43. Medication errors related to potentially dangerous abbreviations. *Sentinel Event Alert* Issue 23, Sep 2001.

44. *ISMP Medication Safety Alert!* 2 May 2001. Web site: www.ismp.org.

45. National Coordinating Council for Medication Error Reporting and Prevention: Recommendations to correct error-prone aspects of prescription writing (adopted 4 Sep 1996). Web site: www.nccmerp.org.

46. Medication safety issue brief 5: Crucial role of therapeutic guidelines. *Hosp Health Netw* 75:65–6, May 2001.

47. Robertson WO: Errors in prescribing. Presented at the Understanding and Preventing Drug Misadventures Conference. Web site: www.ashp.com/public/proad/mederror/prob.html.

48. Lesar TS, Briceland L, Stein DS: Factors related to errors in medication prescribing. *JAMA* 277(4):312–7, 1997.

Protecting Patients from Treatment Delays with Negative Outcomes

Performance of tests, procedures, treatment, or service by clinical staff must be effective, continuous with other care and care providers, safe, efficient, respectful of the patient, and rendered in a timely manner. *Treatment delay* occurs when any of these items is not provided to patients in a time frame required to meet their care needs. Not all treatment delays, therefore, represent patient safety issues. In the best case, such delay may result in inconveniencing individuals and their families. In the worst case, the delay may result in death or serious physical or psychological injury.

Treatment delays represent a different type of system failure. Up to this point, this book has addressed failures that result from some kind of action (a failure of commission). With treatment-delay sentinel events, the failure is the lack of action itself (an omission). Treatment delays represent a failure to provide appropriate care.

The systems established by health care organizations for providing care and services and the ability of staff within the organization to move patients through the health care process are foremost in maintaining timely care. Organization leaders, including medical staff leaders, must identify the needs of the populations served and establish the spectrum of care services that will meet those needs in a timely manner that is consistent with the organization's mission. The system of care for individuals served by the organization includes the following phases:

- Access to the care system;
- Admission to the care system;
- Care within the system; and
- Discharge from the care system.

Physicians are integrally involved in each of these phases. Many factors associated with each of these phases can impede the timely completion of care.

Cause for Concern

Data from the Joint Commission's sentinel event database, including more than 1,600 sentinel events reviewed by the organization from January 1995 through May 2002, indicate that delay in treatment accounted for 5.3% of sentinel events, representing the fifth most common type of sentinel event reviewed by the organization.

While hospital EDs are the source of just over one-half of all *reported* cases of patient death or permanent injury due to delays in treatment, Joint Commission sentinel event data reveal that such serious problems can occur in any hospital unit, as well as in other health care settings.[1] Of the 55 reported cases of delays in treatment, 29 were ED related, and 26 cases originated in hospital ICUs, medical–surgical units, inpatient psychiatric hospitals, freestanding and hospital-based ambulatory care services, ORs, and home care settings. Of the 55 reported cases of delays in treatment, 52 resulted in patient death.

The reported reasons for delays in treatment are many and varied. The most common factors are

- misdiagnosis (42%);
- delayed test results (15%);
- physician availability (13%);
- delayed administration of ordered care (13%);
- incomplete treatment (11%);
- delayed initial assessment (7%);
- patient left unattended (4%);
- paging system malfunction (2%); and
- unable to locate ED entrance (2%).

Of the 23 cases involving misdiagnoses, the most frequently missed diagnosis was meningitis (7 cases); 6 of the 7 cases were in children. Other missed diagnoses included various forms of cardiac disease, pulmonary embolism, trauma, asthma, neurological disorder, and four cases of unknown diagnosis because the patient left without being evaluated. Of the 5 cases that occurred in inpatient psychiatric hospitals, all were related to the delayed diagnosis or treatment of nonbehavioral medical conditions.

The Physician's Role

Physicians play a primary role in diagnosing disease and initiating treatment and, thus, in preventing treatment delays with negative outcomes. In ambulatory care settings, physicians and/or physician-led health care teams need to be able to promptly see patients in need of emergency treatment. Patient care schedules must be able to accommodate emergencies requiring speedy assessment and diagnosis by the physician. Then the physicians must diagnose the patient's illness accurately and initiate the proper treatment. In hospitals, long term care facilities, behavioral health care facilities, and other health care settings, the unavailability of physicians—particularly the required physician specialists—can result in treatment delays with negative outcomes.

Misdiagnosis or delayed diagnosis in all health care settings represents a major concern for physicians and is an issue of national importance. In the current litigious medical–legal environment, plaintiffs are garnering an increasing proportion of victories in diagnosis-related malpractice claims.

The recovery rate for plaintiffs increased to 37% in 2000 from 31% in 1999, according to data from Jury Verdict Research.[2] "Medical care is not an exact science and an individual's clinical judgment is not always perfect. Most people, certainly most juries, understand fallibility," comments one writer.[3] Given the time constraints and other challenges of contemporary medical practice, mistakes and treatment delays resulting in negative outcomes occur.

Common Systems Failures

The causes of sentinel events due to delays in treatment cross disciplinary boundaries and reflect systems failures. Organizations experiencing treatment delay–related sentinel events reviewed by the Joint Commission to date identified the following as root causes:

- Inadequate communication among caregivers, most often with or between physicians;
- Inadequate patient assessment;
- Discontinuity of care across care settings and other continuum of care issues;
- Inadequate availability of critical patient information;
- Insufficient staff orientation and training;
- Insufficient staffing levels; and
- Lack of available physician specialists.

A chart illustrating the percentage of treatment delay sentinel events attributed to each root cause appears as Figure 5-1, page 89. For most failures, multiple causes were identified. Among the ED cases, the most commonly cited root causes were staffing (34%) and availability of physician specialists (21%); overcrowding was cited as a contributing factor in 31% of the cases.

According to an April 2002 American Hospital Association survey of hospitals,[4] more than 90% of large hospitals (300 or more beds) reported having EDs at or over operating capacity. And, according to the survey, capacity constraints translate into longer waiting times for treatment, longer stays in the ED,

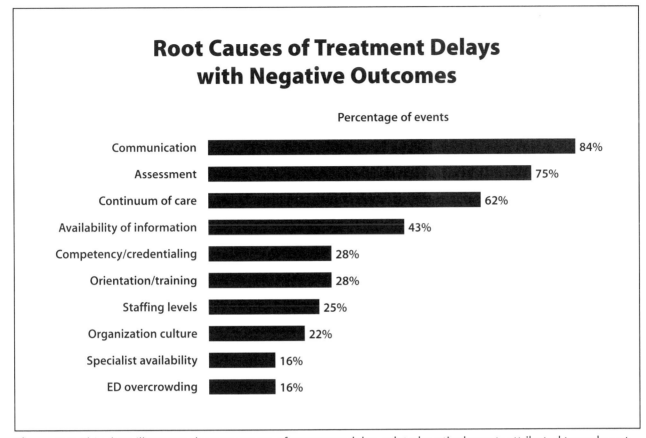

Figure 5-1. This chart illustrates the percentage of treatment delay–related sentinel events attributed to each root cause. For most sentinel events, multiple causes were identified.

and longer waiting times to get admitted to a general acute, critical care, or psychiatric bed.

"Delays have always been a source of concern for emergency departments, due in part to the inability to turn people away," says Michael Rapp, past president of the American College of Emergency Physicians. "Providing timely treatment and avoiding delays is a constant challenge. Causes of delays tend to be multi-factorial, and both external and internal to the emergency department. Currently, issues of overcrowding are a threat to emergency departments everywhere, frequently stemming from insufficient inpatient beds. Other external factors can include slow turnaround of lab and X-ray results."[1]

A thorough look at the root causes and responsibilities of physicians as team members is critical to the successful development and implementation of effective failure prevention strategies. The remainder

of this chapter focuses on prevention strategies physicians can use when working in a team environment to help reduce the likelihood of treatment delay–related deaths and injuries.

System Solution 1: Communication

Sentinel Event Example 1: Misuse of Orders

A frail elderly woman with a fast and thready pulse is admitted to the hospital from a long term care facility. The admitting physician is worried that the woman's dosage of digoxin, one of several cardiac medications the woman is receiving, may not have been sufficient to strengthen her heartbeat and prevent pulmonary edema. The physician orders a digoxin level to be drawn with the afternoon laboratory values. The nurse misses the order on the admission order form and does not include an order for a digoxin level on the slip provided to the laboratory phlebotomist drawing the woman's blood.

The physician visits the woman during rounds that night. He notes rales during ascultation of the woman's breath sounds and that the woman appears to be more congested. The physician makes a mental note to check the digoxin level because the woman's pulse is weak and fast. When reviewing the woman's clinical record, the physician does not see the results of the ordered digoxin level and assumes that it was an oversight on his part. He orders another digoxin level to be drawn in the morning and also orders 40 mg of Lasix. The physician did not order digoxin to be given when the woman arrived earlier in the day, and he did not order digoxin to be administered when he saw her later that night.

The nurse caring for the woman on the evening shift removes the orders for the blood draw in the morning and does not review the record for outstanding orders for previous blood specimens. The nurse on the day shift when the woman was admitted also did not review the pending laboratory tests, which would have indicated the fact that the digoxin level was not drawn. The patient receives 40 mg of Lasix and appears to be breathing a little more easily. The report to the night shift nurse states that the woman appeared to have some labored respiration, which resolved with Lasix.

At about 2:00 AM, the woman becomes very short of breath and is clearly in pulmonary edema. The nurse on the night shift telephones the resident on call to visit the woman. The resident evaluates the woman and reviews the record, noting that a digoxin level was ordered when the woman was admitted and that the results were not in the record. He asks the nurse why the results were not obtained. The night nurse calls the laboratory. Laboratory staff state that they did not receive a slip for the earlier draw but that the woman is on the morning roster for digoxin levels. They suggest that if the physician is concerned, the physician ask for the results "stat." They also indicate that digoxin levels cannot be run on the off-shift hours.

The resident appears satisfied with that explanation and orders more Lasix, reduces the IV fluid volume rate, and leaves the unit. The woman diureses, improves slightly,

and breathes through the night. The levels are drawn the next morning, but the results are not requested stat. The day shift nurse does not follow up on the status of the results, which indicate insufficient digoxin levels. The results are filed in the woman's record without action.

At about noon, the woman experiences cardiac arrest and cannot be resuscitated. The attending physician is informed that the woman has expired. He comes to the nurses' station to fill out the death certificate. Reviewing the woman's record, he realizes that the first digoxin level was not drawn. The value from the morning draw indicates that the cause of death is directly related to the lack of digoxin. The physician calls the hospital's risk manager to express concern about treatment delays.

Sentinel Event Example 2*: Ineffective Communication

Following complaints of an episode of diarrhea, nausea, and cramping abdominal pain, a 72-year-old man was seen at his internist's office at approximately 5:00 PM. An abdominal exam revealed tenderness that was somewhat diffuse below his umbilicus, but rebound tenderness was not present. No positive findings were noted on rectal exam, but an abdominal x-ray demonstrated large amounts of stool with question of impaction. The white blood cell count was normal. The patient was discharged with a probable diagnosis of gastroenteritis. Compazine and a Fleet enema were prescribed with oral instructions to seek emergency care if he experienced increased abdominal pain or fever.

At 1:00 AM, the patient's wife called the after-hours emergency line to report that her husband was experiencing intermittent, knife-like pain in his right shoulder and right lower chest. This call was answered by a physician's assistant (PA) who had on-line access to the internist's notes from the earlier visit and reassured her that the pain was probably related to the gastritis. The PA advised the patient's wife to give her husband a

---

*   Source: Schaefer M: Closed claim abstract: Delay in emergency hospitalization. Forum *18(3)*, Oct 1997. Used with permission of the Risk Management Foundation of the Harvard Medical Institutions.

Compazine suppository. Following this exchange, the patient's wife claims she said, "Thank you, doctor."

The patient's wife called again at 5:30 AM to report that her husband passed out following administration of the enema. This call was answered by the same PA, who advised that her husband was probably reacting to the Compazine and the enema. He advised her to keep her husband in bed, have him sip clear liquids, and to call his physician at 8:00 AM.

A third call was placed at 5:51 AM by the patient's wife to the same PA to report that her husband had fallen in the bathroom and could not get up. She was again advised that her husband was just having a reaction to the Compazine. At this time, the PA authorized an ED visit. Three minutes later she called to report that her husband had passed out and was unresponsive. The PA ordered an ambulance. Upon arrival by the emergency technicians, the patient was in cardiac arrest and was pronounced dead shortly after admission.

Autopsy revealed that the patient had previously undiagnosed rectal cancer which caused the colon to rupture and a cardiac arrest. Extensive coronary artery disease was also noted.

Adequate and effective communication among caregivers is critical to the provision of high-quality care and the prevention of sentinel events related to treatment delays. In the first example, communication was inadequate on a number of fronts. The physician should have ordered a hold on the digoxin dose for that morning, until the levels were received, and then suggested a call for advice on appropriate dosing. The physician might have left dosing parameters for the nurse to follow, dependent on the levels of digoxin in the woman's blood. In that case, the nurse would have been able to make an appropriate calculation of the dose or determine if the dose needed to be withheld and the level reevaluated. The night nurse had a responsibility to communicate the pending laboratory results that would affect the woman's medication. The day

nurse had a responsibility to review the pending laboratory results and adjust the woman's medication schedule. The day nurse could have held the digoxin until the lab values were received and then called the physician for a dose adjustment. Laboratories must flag unusual or significant test results in a manner that will draw attention to the findings.

Too often, staff seek out overly simple solutions to such communication failures, for example, by having all individuals receive digoxin in the afternoon when lab test results are generally available. If the nursing staff do not understand the rationale of this practice, errors may occur.

In the second example, the physician assistant did not follow approved telephone protocols for handling after-hours telephone triage. She should have identified herself by name and title to the patient and ensured that the patient and family were clear that they were not speaking to a physician.

 Work with administrative and medical staff to develop and implement effective procedures for contacting on-call specialists. Respond to requests promptly. Prompt communication with on-call specialists is critical to an organization's ability to protect patients from treatment delays with negative outcomes. For example, an ED physician needs to rely on specialists such as trauma surgeons, neurologists, and cardiac surgeons to provide timely care to individuals presenting in the ED with gunshot wounds, strokes, and heart attacks. On-call physicians must be reachable via pager, phone, or other electronic means and must be provided with the critical information that will help them gauge the urgency of the patient care need. Treatment prioritization among patents is often required.

 Ensure effective communication of information related to patient needs from one physician to the next and from the medical to nursing staff and vice versa. Physicians need to establish and implement workable communication systems to transmit information from one caregiver to the next and, in some cases, from one health care organization to the next. In-person reports and written documentation are most effective. Tape-recorded reports, although commonly used as a backup mechanism by nursing staff, do not provide the opportunity for the incoming caregivers to ask questions of the previous caregivers. It is imperative that the physician and nurse beginning to care for an individual receive all the required information at the start of care. Nurses can document critical elements on forms developed to capture important information that must be communicated to the next team or shift. Such forms help to ensure that the nurse communicates necessary information during the verbal report to the attending physician and nursing colleagues.

JCAHO recommends physician participation in implementing processes and procedures designed to improve the timeliness, completeness, and accuracy of staff-to-staff communication, including communication with and between resident and attending physicians.

 Respond promptly and appropriately to critical information received from other disciplines. Prompt ordering of appropriate treatment by physicians is dependent on information from nursing and other staff working in hospital, ambulatory, long term care, home care, and behavioral health care organizations. All staff must know how to process information critical to patient safety and other outcomes appropriately. For instance, in the first examples, the nurse should know to call the woman's physician with the test results. A system of "panic value" reporting must be implemented to flag abnormal results received from laboratories. Physicians must respond promptly to critical information.

 Establish protocols for communication with the patient and family members. Ensure staff competence and compliance. Office-based physicians and physicians with staff in

health care organizations need to establish telephone protocols for staff use for communicating with patients and family members. The protocol should cover when consultation with a supervising physician is required and the required components of documentation, such as the date, time of the call, patient's complaints, and any advice given.[5]

 Reduce reliance on verbal orders and require a procedure of read back or verification when verbal orders are necessary. As described in Chapter 4, verbal orders increase the probability of miscommunication of information that is critical to patient safety. In the limited number of instances in which verbal orders are necessary, physicians should require those receiving the orders to read back the entire orders.

System Solution 2: Assessment

Sentinel Event Example: Inadequate Assessment

An 87-year-old woman with urosepsis enters an ED at 8:00 AM and is evaluated by an ED nurse. The woman is frail and diaphoretic and has a fever of 102.6°F. She is admitted to the hospital. The nurse places the woman's record in the box outside the woman's room, indicating a priority designation in order to call the ED physician's attention to the woman's condition. Anticipating the need for IV therapy, the nurse starts a peripheral line.

Approximately 15 minutes later, the ED physician comes into the room, reviews the record briefly, and determines that the woman may be septic. When contemplating antibiotic treatment for urosepsis in an elderly person, it is appropriate to order renal function tests and await the results before administering antibiotics. The physician confirms the need for an IV line and orders renal function tests and a chest x-ray. There is a delay in the renal function testing. There is also a delay in the nursing and medical staff's initial assessment of the woman. Both delays are the result of staffing shortages. An hour and a half elapses before the woman receives a physical examination by the ED physician, at approximately 11:00 AM.

Two hours after she enters the ED, the woman's renal function tests have not been completed. The ED physician orders intravenous antibiotics to be given every 6 hours, pending the test results, and refers the woman to her attending physician for admission. The nurse in the ED makes the necessary arrangements to admit the woman. Another hour elapses before the woman is admitted to the 40-bed medical–surgical unit. The woman is received by a nurse on that unit and placed in a bed. Meanwhile, her renal test results are received, indicating a need for antibiotic therapy. The orders for IV antibiotics sit in the ED for an hour before they are transcribed and the pharmacy receives the order. Pharmacy staff deliver the antibiotics and place them in the medication room, noting the administration times of 10:00 AM, 4:00 PM, 10:00 PM, and 4:00 AM.

The woman's vital signs are taken at 2:00 PM, at which point, she has been in the care setting for 6 hours. Her temperature has increased and is now 103.2°F. The nurse administers acetaminophen per order of the house officer. When the nurse comes into the room with the first dose of the woman's antibiotics at 3:45 PM, the woman is comatose and unresponsive. She is in septic shock. She is promptly transferred to the ICU, where she dies 12 hours later, after having received only one dose of antibiotics.

This example illustrates the interaction of numerous root causes that contributed to a sentinel event, including inadequate communication, lack of information availability, inadequate continuity of care, and inadequate assessment, the latter of which is addressed in this section.

EDs are very busy places in many communities and, often, the adequacy of staffing is an issue. Delays in treatment constitute a serious problem in such an environment. The medical and nursing staff should have assessed the woman promptly and reassessed

her to track her increased fever. Assessments must be completed within the time frame specified by organization policy. Thorough assessment helps to ensure proper treatment. The woman in this example should have received antibiotics as soon as there was a reasonable certainty that she was septic or had the potential to become septic. The orders for antibiotics should have been clearly written for immediate administration. This lacking, the woman went to the medical–surgical unit, where the routine protocol for medication administration was followed.

Each discipline is responsible for recommending the number of staff necessary to complete assessments in a timely fashion. Leaders are responsible for maintaining safe staffing levels that will ensure care timeliness. This is critical. For example, delay in recognition of a laboring mother's prolapsed cord in a busy labor and delivery suite could mean the difference between life and death for a fetus in delivery. Monitoring the fetus's heart rate ensures that the mother's contractions are productive and not destructive to the fetus.

The Joint Commission developed a new staffing effectiveness standard that became effective for accredited hospitals in July 2002. Accredited hospitals must select two human resources indicators (for example, overtime, staff injuries, on call or per diem use) and two clinical/service screening indicators (for example, falls, length of stay, pneumonia) to assess staffing effectiveness and identify staffing needs.

Prevention Strategy *Perform an initial medical assessment in a timely manner.* Prompt assessment helps to ensure prompt diagnosis and treatment in all care settings. EDs present particular challenges to timeliness. In the example above, it is likely that the ED nurse was following a policy that treatment is not conducted in the ED but relegated to nursing staff in medical–surgical units. Physician and nurse leaders must address this policy. Because there are limited personnel in many EDs, moving patients through the ED and into care units becomes imperative. This can be a challenge if hospital beds are not available. It may not be entirely clear that a dose of antibiotics could save a life, but it has been well established that urinary tract infections and pneumonia in elderly, compromised individuals can lead to septicemia and serious failure of body systems in a relatively short period of time.

In an earlier example in this chapter, the physician should not have relied solely on the findings and treatment of a previous treating physician. A hands-on exam and evaluation by the physician reduces the risk of a treatment delay or misdiagnosis.

 Ensure staffing and training necessary to perform assessments in a timely fashion. Staffing adequacy and timely assessments go hand in hand. Consider the scenario of the prolapsed cord. Obstetric residents and interns in teaching hospitals can perform a digital examination to assess the position of the baby and the potential for a prolapsed cord. Staff in a community hospital in which there are fewer deliveries needs to be trained at a different level. Physicians can work with medical staff and other organization leaders to identify staffing and training issues related to assessment that could compromise patient safety.

 Reassess regularly to monitor care interventions. Appropriate care involves regularly reassessing the patient's response to care. Delays in reassessing or monitoring an individual can lead to adverse occurrences. For example, continuously monitoring a woman in labor in the delivery suite is imperative. As the stages of labor progress and delivery comes closer, the potential for difficulty increases. The required staff-to-patient ratio changes as the woman progresses through labor. Problems can arise, especially with women who have not had sufficient prenatal care and hence may have latent problems that are not evident or anticipated. The physician must be summoned at exactly the right time, a point that is

often difficult to determine, as labor progresses. In organizations in which there are no house staff, nursing staff need to make that decision independently. Usually, criteria have been developed by medical and nursing staff to allow for a consistent decision mechanism.

Inadequate monitoring and reassessment contributed to the sentinel event described previously for the 87-year-old woman with sepsis. With severely compromised individuals, physicians and nurses must recognize the signs of decompensation and increasing illness. They must evaluate the individual's present condition, compare it to the past reported condition, and apply principles of critical thinking and deductive reasoning to determine care needs.

System Solution 3: Information Management

Sentinel Event Example: Lack of Follow-up

A 75-year-old man who had triple vessel bypass surgery a month ago is accepted for home care by a visiting nurses association (VNA). The local medical center's discharge-planning department reports that the man's care will be quite involved. He is a diabetic who does not comply with dietary recommendations. He has only marginal circulation in his lower extremities, is at risk for stroke, and is on a host of medications that will require close monitoring. The man's wife is disabled and cannot contribute to her husband's care or oversight.

The man's medications include warfarin, a drug used to thin the blood and decrease the likelihood of clot formation, and Tegretol, a drug used in some instances as a mild analgesic, with specific neurological advantages for trigeminal neuralgia. These two drugs interact to increase (potentiate) anticoagulation. International Normalized Ratio (INR) is one of the tests for reduced clotting factors. A normal INR is 1. The decreased clotting factor that generally is desired is between 2 to 3, meaning that it takes blood about twice the time to clot in an adequately treated patient. Regulation of medication doses is critical. An INR of 4 to 7 could lead to bleeding that could go beyond superficial bruising and actually affect vital organs, including the brain, bowel, heart, and so forth.

The VNA receives a copy of the man's discharge summary and a copy of the interagency referral form. The information is limited. The VNA also receives the name of a primary care physician who has been assigned to the man's care and has seen him only once while he was in the hospital. After the first visit to the man's home, a nurse reviews the medications and helps him organize a pill dispenser so that he knows what to take in the morning, at midday, and at night for seven days. The VNA nurse will visit the man on Tuesdays, Thursdays, and Saturdays. On the Tuesday of the second week, the nurse draws blood samples and delivers them to the laboratory. The physician's office receives the results, showing an INR of 5.5. The physician files the results and does not act on them.

A week goes by and the visiting nurse, having complied with his responsibility, does not check with the physician's office for the laboratory results, assuming that they were probably in order. If there had been a problem, the nurse reasons that the physician would have phoned new orders to the pharmacy and notified him. On Thursday, the nurse goes to the man's home and finds no one there. The man had been admitted to the hospital after collapsing at home the night before. The nurse travels to the hospital and locates the man's wife in the ICU waiting room, surrounded by distraught family members. The man is on a ventilator in the ICU, fully obtunded, and in a vegetative state. He suffered a stroke. The nurse manager of the ICU informs the VNA nurse that the man's bleed was due to a significantly elevated prothrombin time, with an INR of 7.

Clearly, the attending physician had a responsibility to contact the visiting nurse with the results of the INR. The nurse had as much responsibility to follow up nonforthcoming results with a call to the physician's office. For a patient such as the man described in this example, vigilance and oversight are

very important. The man did not have enough information to question the results, and his wife was not able to help in managing his treatment. The man required education on the association of Tegretol and warfarin and the probability of their potentiating effects. The delayed review of pending results and the failure to address information that was critical to the man's care compromised the care provided and resulted in a fatal bleed.

Individuals frequently require care across multiple care settings. If physicians or other caregivers lack critical information about a patient, treatment delays and incorrect treatment decisions can occur.

The transmission of data and information must be timely and accurate. In addition, the information must be acted on to meet patient needs. If information is not transmitted at a time of critical value or managed and acted upon appropriately by health care professionals, treatment can be delayed. Treatment could also be delayed when

- information retrieval systems do not allow off-shift staff to access information;
- ambulatory and emergency information are not part of the retrieval system;
- information is not stored in a central location; and
- information is not tracked, and therefore the clinical record may not be present and its location may be unknown.

The patient's clinical record, logs that are kept on the unit, and computer screens that trigger the viewer to address pending test results are all information management systems that support the individual's care and help reduce the likelihood of treatment delays. If these systems fail to prompt an action on the part of the responsible caregiver, their efficacy has in some way been compromised.

Laboratory test results are communicated to care settings in a number of ways. Some organizations have a computerized system that notes the results on the record as soon as they are obtained in the laboratory. In some such circumstances, staff may miss noting critical values. Or, if the system requires the ordering physician to look up results from a terminal in the hospital, results may be missed entirely until some adverse event occurs. In many instances, laboratories call care units if the critical values (sometimes called "panic" values) are grossly out of range. If for any reason the laboratory cannot reach a staff member on the nursing unit or if the laboratory technologist speaks with a staff member who forgets to communicate the value, the information may sit on the patient's record and be noted too late to be appropriately addressed.

Physicians should be part of the process of developing and implementing appropriate information and communication systems. Systems should address issues such as how information systems can be improved to call critical aspects of care to the attention of medical and nursing staff when medication and laboratory values must be correlated and how abnormal lab or radiology results should be communicated.

The examples in this chapter illustrate the critical importance of timely and thorough information management and, as discussed earlier, complete caregiver communication.

 Document care provided and response to care. Timely completion of clinical records is critical to quality care and to the prevention of sentinel events related to treatment delays. Physicians must document the care they order and provide, as well as the individual's response to care. The clinical record is frequently a complex and confusing communication tool. However, documentation of care in the clinical record is often a primary method used by caregivers to communicate information. Therefore, it is essential. If information is received and filed in the record without being addressed or acted on by the appropriate individual, the information is as good as

lost. In such cases, information management certainly has fallen short of expectations and the purposes for which the record was designed.

 Act in a timely and appropriate manner on information received. Clinical records must be designed in a way that ensures that information filed in the record is seen and acted on by the appropriate individual(s). This includes information about the results of tests. If the record shows that a test has been ordered and obtained, there must be a system to match the results with that order for the test. In all settings, physicians work with nurses to ensure that this happens. Records should include a section that addresses pending results. Physicians and their staff should have computerized or manual reminder systems to check on follow-up tests, appointments, and so forth. Sidebar 5-1, page 97, provides numerous follow-up strategies.

When home care providers perform tests on individuals, the results most likely go to the ordering physician. The laboratory performing the test should either place a flag on the report to the physician's office, suggesting follow-up with the visiting nurse, or the laboratory should be encouraged to send a copy of the test results to the home care agency for inclusion in its files. The ordering physician is responsible for communicating test results to the patient and family.

At times, the failure of secondary communication, such as communication between treating physicians and consulting physicians, can contribute to treatment delay. "In the face of persistent symptoms, over-reliance on verbal or preliminary reports of radiology or laboratory findings may miss important differential clues that a dialogue among clinicians would have identified," notes one expert.[6]

 Ensure availability of the clinical record. Clinical records must be available to all those who require the information in order to provide safe and timely care. Many

Sidebar 5-1. Keeping Track of Test Results and Return Appointments

In the course of a busy practice, physicians frequently lose track of important test results that may significantly affect diagnosis and treatment. Often, physicians will ask patients to call back to report on their status or to check on test results. Still, the provider remains responsible if the patient fails to do so and an untoward result ensues.

Two simple "low-tech" techniques to avert misadventures, such as failure to diagnose, include:

- create a file of index cards by dates. At the end of the clinical encounter, jot down the patient's name, test or clinical situation of concern, the dates of encounter, and when results or contact are due;
- review your patient schedule at the end of the day with charts in hand; see which patients need follow-up in regard to test results or appointments; create the index cards as noted above.

Then, each morning review your index file by date.

An alternate method is to enter the data in your personal digital assistant (PDA). Still, the index file may be quicker!

It is more difficult to keep track of patients who are of concern and who should return at a later date. If your scheduling module extends for three or more months, do have patients make the appointment on exiting the office. This way, you will have a record available to send reminders and follow-up on no-shows.

Keep in mind that appointments made long in advance result in more missed or canceled appointments, and these require follow-up again on their own!

Source: Frenkel M: Keeping track of test results and return appointment. *J Med Pract Manage* 17:57, Sep/Oct 2001. Used with permission.

organizations are considering or implementing electronic record systems, which help ensure the availability of up-to-date clinical records and can permit access from multiple locations. "In the office practice setting, the paper record covers care provided there, but contains little information pertaining to care outside the office practice (for example, ED visits, or discharge summaries)," notes one risk management expert. "A computer-based patient record can bridge current medical information needs at any site. This reduces the potential for incorrect decisions and improves healthcare in general."[6]

System Solution 4: Orientation and Training

Sentinel Event Example: Unclear Communication

A 60-year-old woman goes to an ambulatory care clinic to receive her annual physical from her long-time physician. The physician gives the woman a prescription for an annual mammogram, which she schedules for two weeks later. Following the mammogram, the woman is informed by a member of the diagnostic testing staff that there are "problems" with the test and that she will hear from her physician's office. A week later, a nurse in the physician's office calls the woman and informs her that additional mammogram views are required. The nurse does not express the physician's wish that the tests be done immediately or that there is a potential health problem. Required to perform extra duties because of short staffing, the nurse files the x-ray reports in the woman's medical record rather than in the proper file for tests requiring follow-up.

The woman does not forget the need for a follow-up mammogram and calls the physician's office to ascertain whether a repeat mammogram has been ordered. Another office employee assumes that if the woman did not get a call from the physician directly, the woman has nothing to worry about and should relax. The woman does not question the employee's answer or tell the employee about the nurse's call, and she attempts to think no more about it.

Several weeks later, the woman calls the physician's office again, noting that she can feel a hard lump in her breast and mentioning that it hurts. The physician tells her to come into the office right away. Upon review of her record, the physician finds the results and orders another mammogram with needle localization "stat." The woman has the test, which identifies a change in the size of a nodule from a previous mammogram. This requires an immediate biopsy, which is positive for cancer. Subsequent surgery reveals that the cancer has metastasized.

This example illustrates the critical link between staff training, staffing levels, and the provision of timely treatment. All health care organizations and physicians working in office-based settings frequently struggle with the challenge of maintaining adequate staffing in times of increasing care loads. Staff positions may be reevaluated and staff members cross-trained to work in multiple areas. Physicians must ensure that their staffs are trained to flag abnormal tests results and promptly bring them to the physicians' attention.

All practitioners have preferences for the particular way that data, including test results, are processed.

In the case of the woman in the example, the practitioner's procedure for processing test results was not followed by the newly cross-trained nurse. Cross-trained staff must be thoroughly trained in procedures and protocols and ask questions about procedures to use when there is an unusual situation, such as abnormal test findings. Organizations should also consider standardizing the procedure used to process data, including test results, so that all practitioners follow the same procedure. This would free nurses from having to recall the different preferences of each practitioner.

Insufficient staffing levels also could have contributed to the delay in the woman's treatment. Care areas must be adequately staffed to assess and care for individuals. Staff scheduling can be a problem during holidays and off-shifts or following dramatic increases in the census. Physicians should help ensure that staff case loads and responsibilities allow for the effective and timely collection of all information needed to care for individuals adequately.

Prevention Strategy ***Ensure staff competence.*** Physicians and leaders in health care organizations must ensure that the competence and quality of all staff members are continually assessed and improved. According to the procedures established by the medical practice in the example, the nurse was responsible for identifying the presence of a problem in the test results (that is, a possible tumor) and bringing the study results to the physician's attention. Procedures for doing so include presenting all test results to the physician at a scheduled time of day so that the physician can review them and determine what action needs to be taken. Physicians train their staff to recognize common negative and positive results requiring the physicians' attention. The physician is responsible for ensuring that a call is made to the patient. Even if the study results are entirely negative, under normal operating procedure, nursing staff should make the physician aware of the results. The physician would then direct an office staff member or nurse to call the patient.

Prevention Strategy

Help to ensure safe staffing levels.
Leaders need to ensure that physicians and nurses are able to care for individuals in a timely and effective manner. With the previous example in mind, this means having time to evaluate the laboratory and x-ray results received in the office. In this scenario, insufficient staffing may have hindered timely notification of test results to the physician. Scheduling time for review of laboratory and radiographic results is critical. This can be performed at the end of the day to ensure receipt of the maximum number of test results. If results are pending for tests that were performed or ordered that day, there should be a procedure to hold the record out of the file for follow-up at a subsequent time. If the record is filed away at the end of the work day, a tickler system could alert the office staff that test results are pending and that they need to be followed up on if not received within a set period of time. For example, mammograms may be read only on Tuesdays and Thursdays in some smaller organizations, although they could be performed daily. The office staff need to know when a reasonable time frame for receipt of test results has been exhausted and when follow-up is required. Processes should be designed to minimize variation, which increases the likelihood of error.

Closing Comments

In each phase of care, many opportunities exist for systems to break down, leading to delays in treatment that result in negative outcomes for patients. Delays in testing and obtaining test results, delays in implementing care guidelines, and delays with the performance and documentation of H&Ps, and assessments can corrupt the process of establishing care priorities based on identified needs. These delays can lead to unexpected and adverse consequences. As patient care leaders, physicians are well positioned to help reduce the likelihood of untoward events resulting from treatment delays.

REFERENCES

1. Joint Commission: Delays in treatment. *Sentinel Event Alert* Issue 26, 17 Jun 2002.
2. Jury Verdict Research: Medical malpractice verdict and settlement study released (press release). Horsham, PA: Jury Verdict Research, 22 Mar 2002.
3. Sarrouf C: Narrow diagnostic focus: A plaintiff attorney's perspective. *Forum* 18:15, May 2002.
4. *Emergency Department Overload: A Growing Crisis.* The Results of the American Hospital Association Survey of Emergency Department (ED) and Hospital Capacity, Apr 2002. Web site: www.msha.com/press/pdf_files/MSHA_ED_Presentation.pdf.
5. Schaefer M: Closed claim abstract: Delay in emergency hospitalization. *Forum* 18(3), Oct 1997.
6. Dwyer K: Multiple systems breakdowns. *Forum* 21:19, Summer 2001.

PROTECTING PATIENTS FROM SERIOUS INJURY OR DEATH IN PHYSICAL RESTRAINTS

Every health care organization strives to provide effective, efficient care in a safe environment and with respect for the rights and dignity of the individuals receiving care. The use of restraint and seclusion represents one of the most complex issues in clinical care—one requiring a delicate balance between safety and rights.

Whereas practitioners traditionally saw as a necessary intervention option in order to protect those in their care from injuries and possibly death, many practitioners and patients now recognize that physical restraint is dangerous and can do more harm than good. When used improperly, restraint can lead to increased length of stay, serious complications related to immobility, the violation of individual rights, and death or serious injury.

The best way to avoid such risk is to *not* use restraint. At times, however, when other interventions are not effective or appropriate, restraint or seclusion may be the only possible alternative to prevent harm to the individual or other persons or to ensure a safe treatment environment.

The Joint Commission defines a *physical restraint* as any method of physically restricting a person's freedom of movement, physical activity, and normal access to the body.[1] This encompasses many physical devices, such as wrist restraints, jacket vests, and mitts, as well as physical procedures such as therapeutic or protective holds. Other examples of physical restraints include

- waist restraints or leg restraints that restrict a person's freedom of movement;
- lap buddies, belts, "geri" chairs, or trays that keep the body immobile in a chair and cannot be removed by the patient;
- belts, tightly tucked sheets, or other items that confine individuals to their beds;
- protective or therapeutic holds;
- comfort or safety blankets; and
- all other devices or human actions that restrict an individual's freedom of movement.

For purposes of this discussion, restraint differs from medical immobilization, such as body restraint during surgery, arm restraint during intravenous administration, and temporary physical restraint before administration of electroconvulsive therapy.[2] These are considered regular parts of such procedures.

In long term care organizations, *restraint* is defined as any method (chemical* or physical) of restricting a resident's freedom of movement, including seclusion and limitation of physical activity or normal access to the body that
- is not a usual and customary part of a medical diagnostic or treatment procedure to which the resident or his or her legal representative has consented;
- is not indicated to treat the resident's medical condition or symptoms; or

---

* For the purposes of this chapter, sentinel events resulting from the use of chemical restraints are not considered restraint-related sentinel events but, rather, medication-related sentinel events, which are covered in Chapter 4.

Sidebar 6-1.
Factors That May Contribute to Increased Risk of Restraint-Related Death

Joint Commission analysis identified the following factors that may contribute to increased risk of death. These include restraining an individual

- who smokes;
- with deformities that preclude the proper application of a restraining device (especially vest restraints);
- in the supine position (may predispose the individual to aspiration);
- in the prone position (may predispose the individual to suffocation); and
- in a room that is not under continuous observation by staff.

Source: Joint Commission: Preventing restraint deaths. *Sentinel Event Alert* Issue 8, 18 Nov 1998.

- does not promote the resident's independent functioning.[2]

Cause for Concern

The FDA estimates that at least 100 deaths result each year from improper use of restraint devices.[3] The actual number of deaths may very well be higher. Although the Safe Medical Devices Act of 1990 requires all hospitals, nursing homes, and acute care facilities to report deaths related to the use of any medical device to the FDA and the manufacturer, many restraint-related deaths may never have been reported anywhere, particularly those involving protective holds. In October 1998, a series of articles appearing in *The Hartford Courant* reported on deaths following use of physical restraint in behavioral health care facilities. A 50-state survey conducted by the Connecticut newspaper revealed at least 142 deaths in the past decade connected with the use of physical restraint or seclusion.[4] Another survey conducted for the newspaper by a research specialist

at the Harvard Center for Risk Analysis estimated that 50 to 150 such deaths may occur each year.

Data from the Joint Commission's sentinel event database indicate that restraint-related deaths and injuries represent 4.6% of all sentinel events reviewed by the Joint Commission between January 1995 and May 2002.[5] Of these 78 deaths and injuries, the majority occurred in psychiatric hospitals, followed by general hospitals, and long term care facilities. In 40% of the cases cited in the Joint Commission's *Sentinel Event Alert*, the cause of death was asphyxiation.[6] Asphyxiation was related to such factors as

- putting excessive weight on the back of the individual in a prone position;
- placing a towel or sheet over the individual's head to protect against spitting or biting; or
- obstructing the airway when pulling the individual's arm across the neck area.

The remaining deaths were caused by strangulation, cardiac arrest, or fire. All the victims of strangulation death were elderly individuals who had been placed in vest restraints. All the victims of death by fire were males who were attempting to smoke or use cigarette lighters to burn off the restraints. Two-point, four-point, or five-point restraints were used in 40% of the cases related to restraint deaths. Therapeutic hold was used in 30% of the cases, restraint vest in 20%, and waist restraint in 10%. Factors identified by Joint Commission staff that may contribute to increased risk of deaths appear in Sidebar 6-1, above.

A review of the literature indicates that organizations with a lower-than-average incidence of violence and of restraint and seclusion use share several key attributes. These appear in Sidebar 6-2, page 103.

Joint Commission Stance

The use of restraint and seclusion has received a great deal of scrutiny during the past two decades. During this period, Joint Commission standards related to restraint and seclusion for JCAHO-accredited organizations have changed to reflect the growing concern of the public, other regulatory bodies, and many health care professionals. The concern is that these interventions are used more often than clinically necessary in all types of health care settings and that they are used in ways that violate individual rights and dignity. The Joint Commission believes that restraint and seclusion are high-risk and problem-prone procedures known to jeopardize the safety of individuals served. As such, JCAHO holds that these procedures should be used only as a last resort.

The Joint Commission's revised restraint and seclusion standards, which became effective January 1, 2001, focus on limiting the use of restraint and seclusion.

In the area of *use of restraint and seclusion*, JCAHO recognizes that restraint and seclusion pose an inherent physical and psychological risk to individuals receiving care and to staff. Their use could also produce other serious consequences such as loss of dignity and violation of an individual's rights. When restraint and seclusion are necessary, trained and competent health care staff should ensure safe use. Restraint and seclusion should be used only in emergencies, when

- risk of harm to the individual or others, including staff, is imminent;
- nonphysical interventions have proven ineffective; or
- safety demands an immediate physical response.

In the area of *reducing the use of restraint and seclusion*, JCAHO indicates that organizations should explore ways to prevent, reduce, and strive to eliminate the use of restraint and seclusion through effective performance improvement initiatives. For some organizations, a restraint-free environment is appropriate to the populations served and clinical services offered and is achievable now or in the future. For other organizations, restraint use may continue to be necessary in clinically justified situations and in the

---

Sidebar 6-2. Key Attributes of Organizations with Lower-Than-Average Incidence of Violence and Restraint and Seclusion Use

- Leaders clearly advocate a treatment philosophy;
- Individuals at risk for violence are identified through assessment on admission to the facility or program;
- Staff are well-trained in aggression management;
- Staff practices encourage maximum use of behavioral modification and de-escalation techniques and minimal use of restraint and seclusion;
- Increased activities for individuals correlate with decreased usage rates of restraints and seclusion;
- The need for restraint or seclusion is based on an evaluation of the individual case and situation; and
- The staff follow guidelines or protocols when restraint or seclusion is indicated.

Source: Joint Commission: *Preventing Adverse Events in Behavioral Health Care: A Systems Approach to Sentinel Events.* Oakbrook Terrace, IL, 1999.

---

foreseeable future, given the organization's populations and clinical services, the current state of knowledge, and available effective alternatives.

JCAHO focuses on the *reason* for restraint and seclusion use rather than the *setting* in which they are used. Staff in all health care organizations should apply the JCAHO requirements based on the reason for restraint and seclusion use. Two major reasons cover all such use:

- *Behavioral health reasons* for the use of restraint or seclusion are primarily to protect the individual against injury to self or others because of an emotional or behavioral disorder. The individual may be receiving care in any type of health care organization.

- *Medical and surgical care reasons* for the use of restraint and seclusion involve directly supporting medical healing, such as protecting a site of care on an individual's body.

None of the requirements apply to standard practices that include limitation of mobility or temporary immobilization related to medical, dental, diagnostic, or surgical procedures and the related postprocedure care processes (for example, surgical positioning, IV armboards, radiotherapy procedures, protection of surgical and treatment sites in pediatric patients); protective equipment such as helmets; adaptive support in response to assessed physical needs of the individual (for example, postural support, orthopedic appliances); and forensic restrictions and restrictions imposed by correction authorities for security purposes.

The Physician's Role

Physicians have ultimate responsibility for overseeing the care provided to individuals in health care organizations. They generally assess individuals for need and type of restraint. "Physicians are in an excellent position to assess patients when the issue of restraints is raised, with the aim of identifying and treating factors contributing to undesirable and high-risk behaviors. This includes reviewing use of inappropriate or excessive medication and screening for pain, infections, metabolic disturbances, and underlying psychiatric conditions," notes one expert team.[7] When restraints are needed, physicians write the orders for them, ensure appropriate use, and review ongoing need for use. In behavioral health settings, psychologists or social workers may also write the orders. Physicians, psychologists, and others must respond appropriately to requests from staff to restrain individuals. They must also maintain open and regular communication with staff who are monitoring an individual in restraint.

Medical leaders and all physicians can be powerful advocates for restraint-free care if they are well informed about factual information related to restraint

alternatives and possible alternative interventions for each individual based on assessed needs. This facilitates a proactive rather than reactive approach to restraint reduction. However, many physicians still believe that they might be sued because of injuries resulting from restraint reduction. Medical leaders can dispel this myth through an educational effort aimed at providing more information and knowledge about the safety and benefits of an incremental risk-taking approach to restraint-free care and education about the risks of restraint use.

Common Systems Failures

Organizations that experienced sentinel events related to restraint use that were reviewed by the JCAHO identified the following root causes[6]:

- Insufficient orientation and training;
- Inadequate patient assessment, including incomplete examination of the individual to identify contraband, such as matches;
- Faulty communication;
- Unsafe equipment or equipment use, such as use of split siderails without siderail protectors; use of two-point rather than four-point restraints; use of a high-neck vest; incorrect application of a restraining device; or a monitor or an alarm not working or not being used when appropriate;
- Inadequate care planning, such as incomplete consideration of alternatives to restraint, restraints used as punishment, and inappropriate room or unit assignments;
- Insufficient staffing levels;
- Lack of needed information; and
- Other factors.

Figure 6-1, page 105, provides a graphic look at the frequency of each type of system failure. A thorough look at common system failures and the responsibilities of physicians as team members is critical to the successful development and implementation of effective failure prevention strategies. The remainder of this chapter focuses on prevention strategies physicians may use when working within a team environment to help reduce the likelihood of deaths or injuries in restraints.

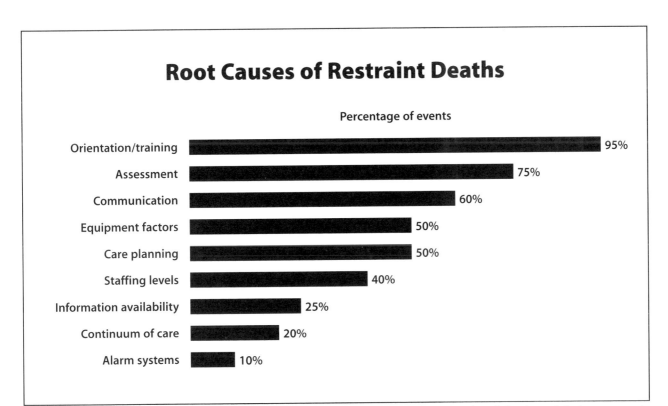

Root Causes of Restraint Deaths

Percentage of events

Orientation/training	95%
Assessment	75%
Communication	60%
Equipment factors	50%
Care planning	50%
Staffing levels	40%
Information availability	25%
Continuum of care	20%
Alarm systems	10%

Figure 6-1. This chart illustrates the percentage of causes at the root of restraint-related deaths or injuries reported to the Joint Commission between January 1995 and May 2002.

System Solution 1: Education, Training, and Restraint-Reduction Advocacy

Sentinel Event Example: Inadequate Training

A temporary staff member is assigned to work in the Alzheimer's unit of a long term care facility. The staff member is not knowledgeable about the application of physical restraint. After working on the unit for less than an hour, the temporary staff member finds one frail and confused resident attempting to climb over his bedrails. The staff member applies the first type of physical restraint that he can find (a vest), without calling the individual's physician for an order. He then continues to care for other residents, neglecting to report use of the vest to the nursing staff.

When a member of the housekeeping staff arrives to provide supplies 45 minutes later, he finds the resident hanging from the restraint, which is attached to the bedrail. The resident is blue and cold and has only a faint pulse. A code is called, and staff attempt to revive

the man. He is placed on a ventilator and admitted to an ICU, but he dies one hour later.

A physician or another LIP must order the use of restraint or seclusion (see pages 115–122). The medical director of the long term care facility described in this example must help ensure that staff receive education and training about alternatives to restraint and training in how to ensure resident safety when restraint is used. During general staff orientation, each staff member must receive basic information regarding restraint use in the organization and alternatives to physical restraint. Clinical staff members should then receive more in-depth information and training and must demonstrate their competence in restraint application and care of individuals in restraints before providing care. Competence assessment can best be accomplished through both written testing and practical application in the education setting before allowing the individual to apply restraints in the clinical setting.

Staff from all shifts as well as part-time and per diem individuals must be included in restraint use orientation, training, and competence assessment programs. Medical, nursing, and allied health students; physicians; nurses; nursing assistants; therapists; and others who may also need to be educated and assessed on restraint policies and procedures should not be overlooked. New staff, agency staff, and staff floated from another area who are not familiar with patients or are not regularly assigned to the unit may cause injury as illustrated in this example. Reassessment of competence must occur regularly, as defined by the organization. Because restraint use is a high-risk area and staff may not frequently use restraint, annual competence assessment is warranted.

Studies have indicated that the commitment and the support of organization leaders, such as medical staff leaders, are absolutely critical to staff training, ongoing education, and competence assessment to reduce restraint and seclusion use and ensure safe use. Leaders can start the educational process of moving toward restraint reduction in their facilities by understanding the staff members' current knowledge levels and attitudes toward the use of restraint and seclusion. Training should address such issues as how physicians with privileges, nurses, and other caregivers view restraint and their roles in restraining or secluding care recipients, their comfort level in managing aggression and other behaviors that commonly lead to restraint or seclusion use, and their knowledge about use of physical restraints and their alternatives.

Physicians' attitudes toward restraint are often critical. If restraint is to be used, physicians must order it. They have the ability to deny staff requests for such use. However, because nurses make the request for restraint use, many studies reported in the literature focus on understanding nurses' attitudes toward restraint use as a first step toward providing appropriate and on-target educational programs. Common myths about the use of restraint and seclusion unfortunately continue to be well entrenched in the minds of many physicians and other health care professionals, patients, families, and the public at large, despite growing scientific and medical evidence debunking such myths. These myths must be dispelled. Physicians can play a major role in this process both individually in how they practice and educationally with staff in health care organizations.

 Dispel the myth that restraint protects individuals from harm and prevents falls and serious injuries, particularly among the frail elderly. Restraint can increase the risk of harm and actually cause harm to individuals. Studies conducted in the long term care community in the 1990s indicate that although the number of falls might have been higher initially in a restraint-free environment, injury severity declined significantly.[8,9,10] Accidental deaths from strangulation or asphyxiation and serious injuries can occur when individuals are trying to escape restraints. Health care professionals commonly believe that asphyxiation occurs chiefly from restraint around an individual's neck. However, it also occurs from constriction of the rib cage. According to Mary Tinetti, director of the Yale Program on Aging, her colleagues, and others, physically restraining older adults can lead to other negative outcomes, such as decubitus ulcers, nosocomial infections, incontinence, loss of functional capacity leading to continued falls and injuries, immobility, cardiac stress, altered nutrition, agitated behaviors, emotional desolation, and feelings of anger, humiliation, discomfort, resistance, and fear.[11,12] Physicians experienced in care of the elderly should be familiar with literature citing such outcomes.

Prevention Strategy *Review the effects of immobility on body systems.* They include the following[3]:
- *Respiratory:* Decreased lung expansion; decreased ciliary movement;
- *Cardiovascular:* Decreased orthostatic competency; increased resting heart rate;
- *Skin:* Increased capillary pressure; increased risk of shear and friction;
- *Musculoskeletal:* Muscle weakness; contracture formation;

- *Urinary:* Decreased gravitational drainage; increased risk of urinary tract infection; increased risk of loss of continence;
- *Gastrointestinal:* Constipation; dehydration; swallowing difficulty; diminished appetite; and
- *Psychological:* Withdrawal; depression; delirium.

Physicians assessing individuals in restraint should be alert to these physiological effects.

 Dispel the myth that restraint use reduces liability risks. Fear of legal liability is one of the most frequently stated reasons for the use of restraint. Physicians and other health care professionals frequently cite threats by the family, such as, "If my parent falls and breaks a bone, I'll sue you," and assume that the family will sue. "It is a common misconception that the legal system will hold healthcare providers liable for patient injury solely because of failure to use restraints," notes one author.[14]

In fact, courts have shown considerable reluctance to hold that a duty to restrain exists. Review of the literature indicates that liability generally results from the use of restraint in an inappropriate manner, rather than from not using physical restraint. The risk of liability for such claims as false imprisonment, assault, and death increases with restraint use. Case law upholds an individual's right to make decisions about his or her health care, including the right to refuse treatment and the right to personal inviolability and dignity. "Failure to restrain a patient, which results in patient injury, is not considered to be negligent. Liability will occur when a particular act or omission on the part of the healthcare provider did not conform to the accepted standard of care, and the deviation from the accepted standard of care harmed the patient," writes one author.[14] Litigation for injuries related to restraint use in acute care settings is more common than litigation for injuries to residents of long term care facilities.

 Dispel the myth that restraint improves an individual's posture and body positioning. As physicians are aware, restraint weakens muscles and discourages the

individual from attempting activities that would improve strength and mobility. Muscles atrophy from lack of exercise, particularly with elderly restrained individuals.

 Dispel the myth that restraint calms an agitated or confused individual and, hence, has therapeutic value. As physicians are aware, the exact opposite is often true. Patients, especially those with cognitive impairments, may become even more agitated when restrained against their will. Their confusion increases because they cannot understand what the restraint is or why it is being applied. Early studies involving long term care residents indicate that cognitively impaired older adults have an increased risk of accidental death because these persons "are less able to understand and cooperate with medical care regimens and may behave in ways that can endanger or disturb patients and staff."[15] Another team describes the confused patient who "may regard a bedrail more as a challenge and scalable height than an impairment to mobility. The resulting fall from the top of a bedrail is much more likely than a simple roll off the bed to cause serious damage."[16]

 Dispel the myth that fewer staff members are required when restraint or seclusion is used, so that use of restraint and seclusion lowers staff costs. Continued use of restraint can lead to an individual's functional decline, requiring more physician and staff time to provide care and services to meet the individual's need and increased length of stay. Individuals who are allowed to ambulate in a safe environment have the opportunity to recover more quickly, resulting in shorter stays. The use of restraint on the basis of staffing patterns for staffing convenience violates federal regulations and JCAHO standards. Two pioneers in the restraint-reduction initiative in long term care facilities, Neville Strumpf and Lois Evans, believe that "organizations" where restraints are justified on the basis [of inadequate staffing] are either so understaffed that minimal standards of care cannot be met, and the facilities should be closed, or staff and administration have not considered the amount of time required for care when restraints are in place, if necessary inspection, release, exercise, toileting, monitoring, and evaluation are to occur."[17] Care provided by interdisciplinary teams and family members can help reduce the cost of providing restraint alternatives. Physicians can take a proactive approach in recommending restraint alternatives.

 Dispel the myth that staff feel more secure and comfortable when restraint is used. Since the early 1980s major studies of the use of restraint have indicated that the opposite is true. Staff interviewed in a psychiatric setting said that the act of restraining caused them to experience feelings of anxiety, inadequacy, frustration, dissatisfaction, being overwhelmed, being drained, and guilt.[18,19] Other studies indicate that staff empathize with individuals who are restrained and recognize that they would not want to be restrained themselves.[19,20] When staff identify and implement alternatives to restraint, their morale, job satisfaction, and pride increase because they are providing high-quality, individualized care. As mentioned earlier, physicians can empower staff by taking a proactive approach to restraint alternatives.

 Dispel the myth that effective alternatives to restraint do not exist. Often health care staff request physicians' order for restraint because they do not know what else to do. This represents an educational, training, and competence challenge for the organizations in which physicians work and a communication challenge for the physicians of whom such requests are made. Highly effective alternatives to restraint use have been described in the professional literature and used in health care organizations for decades. Physicians can educate staff about the risks and limited value of restraints.

A thorough assessment of an individual's needs is critical to identifying and implementing a variety of less restrictive options. As Strumpf and Evans note, "[t]here is no 'magic bullet.' Each [person] and each set of problems must be considered on an individual basis…."[8] This approach is familiar to physicians caring for individual patients. Alternatives may involve changes in care delivery, such as offering exercise programs to patients in acute care settings; environmental management, such as using wrist, bed, or chair alarms and door alarms in behavioral health or dementia units to prevent wandering; physiological alternatives, such as using a percutaneous endoscopic gastrostomy tube, which is rarely disrupted for tube feedings with medical/surgical patients; and psychosocial interventions, such as using behavior modification techniques with individuals who have verbal communication problems and who exhibit aggressive behavior. Table 6-1, pages 109–110, lists devices used as alternatives to siderails.

 Know the alternatives and advocate their use. The professional literature is full of information related to psychosocial, physiological, environmental, and pharmacotherapeutic interventions that can be used appropriately and effectively instead of physical restraint. For example, bed, chair, and door alarms are good alternatives to physical restraint for patients who may wander. Proper pain assessment and management may be needed for some individuals. Increased use of nonmedication alternatives, such as massage therapy, can increase the individual's comfort without compounding symptoms such as mental confusion that could increase the apparent need for restraint use. In some cases, pain medication can be adjusted to decrease hypnotic side effects, drowsiness, and mental confusion. Some organizations also use family members or properly trained "sitters" to stay with the individual as an alternative to restraint use. Physicians should be well versed in restraint alternatives and ready to suggest such alternatives to staff requesting restraint orders.

Sidebars 6-3 and 6-4, pages 111–112, provide numerous other examples of alternatives to restraint.

Table 6-1. Devices Used as Alternatives to Siderails

Device	How Used	Benefits	Risks
Water mattress	When partially filled, this device may reduce movement to edge of the bed.	Lower risk for injury from banging limbs against or climbing over a barrier	May be restrictive for residents with impaired bed mobility
Positioning cushion	Available in several shapes, including wedges and rolls; prevents resident from approaching edge of the bed	Assist in maintaining resident in bed while eliminating risk of banging limbs against rails; easy to remove—can be pushed off bed by resident	May be restrictive for residents with impaired bed mobility
Mats on floor	Soft, thick carpet, cloth, or vinyl covered pads/mats placed around the bed, creating a padded "landing area" during bed-related fall	Nonrestrictive mode; may protect residents from injury if they roll out of bed	Can serve as a tripping hazard for residents and staff; may be an infection control concern as a result of placement on the floor and difficulty with cleaning
Trapeze	Enhances bed mobility by assisting resident in side-to-side turning and raising self up in bed	Nonbarrier alternative	Not practical for cognitively impaired residents who may not respond to teaching or residents with upper extremity mobility limitations
Visual reminders	Signs placed within resident's view that are reminders to use call bell and ask for assistance before getting out of bed	Simple, require little staff time; resident reminded every time sign seen to request help before transferring from bed	May not be effective for visually or cognitively impaired residents
Bedside commode	Placed next to bed when access to the bathroom is not possible	Nonbarrier device; may promote greater independence	May be an infection control concern
Chair or table at bedside	Sturdy chair or table placed at side of bed can be used by resident to help turning and transferring; may provide a proprioceptive cue to the edge of the bed	Readily accessible	Device not "fixed" and may serve as a fall injury hazard
Lower beds	Includes adjustable beds at lowest levels, futon beds, and beds with legs sawed off	Nonbarrier alternative; provide a shorter falling distance and may make transfers easier	Some frail elderly still may be too impaired to make a safe exit attempt. If bed is nonadjustable, a very low bed can be restrictive for residents who have difficulty rising from a low position.
Mattress on the floor	Placed directly on the floor without the bed frame	Nonbarrier alternative; readily accessible; provides a shorter falling distance	May increase risk of back injury to staff; may be restrictive for independently transferring residents who have difficulty rising from the floor

(continued)

Source: Hammond M, Levine JM: Bedrails: Choosing the best alternative. *Geriatr Nurs* 20(6):297–300, Nov–Dec 1999. Used with permission.

Table 6-1. Devices Used as Alternatives to Siderails (continued)

Device	How Used	Benefits	Risks
Alarm device	Alerts staff to resident attempting to exit the bed. Some devices activated by a string clipped to resident's clothing; others placed under or attached to mattress and activated by decreased pressure. All emit an alarm (beep, bell, or even a voice) when the resident attempts to exit the bed. Systems can emit a local alarm or be incorporated into call-bell system.	Nonbarrier mode	Several alarms used on one unit may confuse staff as to which alarm is sounding and where; certain alarms can be deactivated by the resident; if localized at bedside, alarm may distract or frighten resident or roommate; if resident is not assisted immediately, he or she may proceed with unsafe bed-exit attempt; false alarms are common, and staff may become "immune" to sound.
Body padding	Helmets or hip pads to protect against fall-related injuries	Nonbarrier alternative	Can be uncomfortable or embarrassing to wear; may adversely affect skin integrity
Placing bed against the wall	Provides a one-sided barrier	Readily accessible	If bed slides away from wall, resident may fall in between; may violate fire code; encloses one side of the bed and is not to be considered an alternative to bedrails
Half bedrails	Also known as "split" bedrails, take up half the bed length and are adjustable to create several combinations	Easily accessible if bed is equipped with them; can be used as an "enabler" to enhance transfer ability; can serve as a proprioceptive cue	Potential accident hazard, such as banging limbs against, getting stuck in between, or climbing over them
Night light	Provides some light in the room to assist with orientation	Nonrestrictive mode; may serve to prevent unsafe transfers by residents who wake up in the middle of the night	Not useful for visually impaired residents

A recent book from the Joint Commission describes each alternative in full.[21] Physicians who order restraint should try to remain current with alternatives suggested in the literature.

System Solution 2: Assessment

Sentinel Event Example: Incomplete Information

An organization delivering care for postsurgical subacute patients admits a small elderly gentleman at 2:00 PM. The man had a hip replaced three days earlier and still shows signs of confusion. The attending physician orders a waist restraint and the placement of bedrails in the raised position while the man is in bed. The physician is concerned that the man will attempt to walk and bear full weight on the operative hip too soon and possibly cause damage to the new hip prosthesis. The physician notes in her admitting orders that the man is still slightly confused.

Shortly before 3:00 PM, a nursing staff member applies the waist restraint, raises the bedrails as ordered by the physician, and leaves to give a report to

---

Sidebar 6-3. Restraint Alternatives

Alternatives for Managing Aggressive Behavior

- Use de-escalation and other verbal intervention techniques
- Implement behavior modification or token economy programs
- Use time out
- Alter the care environment
- Offer relaxation, exercise, and diversionary activity programs

Alternatives for Maintaining Therapy

- Assess need for therapy and explore therapy alternatives
- Enhance education and communication
- Enlist participation of families and volunteers
- Protect treatment devices
- Modify the environment
- Address physiologic needs
- Use sensors and alarms

Alternatives for Preventing Wandering and Falls

- Offer exercise and ambulation programs
- Meet individual's food, liquid, and toileting needs
- Maximize independence in care
- Promote normal sleep patterns
- Evaluate medications
- Provide effective pain management
- Reassess physical status and review laboratory findings
- Provide for companionship
- Offer diversionary activities
- Reorient individual
- Promote relaxation techniques
- Enhance communication
- Orient individual to care environment
- Ensure safe space layout and clear paths
- Use or modify space to enable close observation of at-risk individuals
- Ensure proper lighting and noise control
- Assure provision and use of proper seating, assistive, and positioning devices
- Assure accessibility of objects of daily living and call lights
- Adapt beds to reduce fall risk
- Adapt or remove siderails

Source: Joint Commission: *Restraint and Seclusion: Complying with Joint Commission Standards.* Oakbrook Terrace, IL, 2002.

the next shift. She fails to indicate in her nursing assessment an increased safety danger due to differences in the type of beds and bedrails used on this unit and the small physical size of the elderly gentleman.

After receiving the report, the nurse on the 3:00 PM to 11:00 PM shift immediately checks the man. She finds him without vital signs, cold, blue, and with his head and neck caught in the larger-size bedrails. Efforts to perform CPR on the man are futile. Less than two hours after admission, he is dead from asphyxiation.

Assessment is an information-gathering and evaluation process. Health care providers collect data about each individual's H&P, psychological status, and social status through initial and ongoing assessment. Analysis of these data yields information vital to meeting the care needs of individuals served. Thorough assessment in effect provides the clues necessary to develop and implement an accurate and complete care plan. At times, clues or their full scope are not readily apparent, and more in-depth assessments are warranted. For example, an initial assessment may

Sidebar 6-4. Strategies to Prevent Line/Tube Removal

IV lines
- Wrap infusion site and arm with stockinette, elastic compression bandage, gauze, or a skin sleeve
- Camouflage the insertion site by using long-sleeved gowns or robes
- Consider using a saline lock (capped IV line) instead of a regular IV line

Urinary catheters
- Discontinue if possible
- Cover or hide catheters with undergarments, apron, or pants
- Place the foley at the foot of the bed and the tube between the individual's legs so that both are out of reach
- Use leg bags if appropriate

Nasogastric tubes
- Consider instead insertion of tube directly into stomach
- Consider using smaller tubes

Abdominal tube
- Use a tube stabilizer
- Cover the insertion site with a loose flextone abdominal binder

Nasal oxygen cannula
- Humidify the oxygen
- Lubricate the individual's nares
- Tape the cannula to the individual's cheeks
- Check the pulse oximetry on room air to assess whether oxygen is still necessary

All
- Use dummy tube to distract care recipient from actual insertion site

Sources: Compiled from Mion LC, Strumpf N: Use of physical restraints in the hospital setting: Implications for the nurse. *Geriatric Nursing* 15:127–32, May/Jun 1994. Mion LC: Establishing alternatives to physical restraint in the acute care setting: A conceptual framework to assist nurses' decision making. *AACN Clinical Issues* 7:592–602, Nov 1996. Rogers PD, Bocchino NL: Restraint-free care: Is it possible? *AJN* 99: 27–33, Oct 1999. Selekman J, Snyder B: Uses of and alternatives to restraints in pediatric settings. *AACN Clinical Issues* 7:603–10, Nov 1996.

indicate that the individual may be at risk for nutritional problems and need detailed assessment by a dietitian. The scope of assessment depends on the individual's diagnosis, the care the individual seeks, the care setting, the individual's response to previous care, and the consent to treatment.

Assessment of individuals at risk for restraint or seclusion generally involves data collection in two areas:
- *Health history:* This might be obtained by medical or nursing staff from interviews of the individual, his or her family, and past care providers and from a review of the individual's clinical record, focusing on such items as medical or behavioral diagnosis(es), relevant medications, and history of falls, aggression, and other behaviors and factors that contribute to at-risk status. Persons aware of the individual's current activities of daily living can provide accurate data; persons from out of town who come in to help address the situation on a short-term basis often are not able to provide accurate information.
- *Physical examination:* Data are obtained by physicians and nursing staff through an examination of the individual, focusing on such factors as cognitive status, blood pressure, pain, sleep, continence, gait, and strength. Assessment of cognitive or behavioral status may require a more in-depth assessment, such as a Mini-Mental Test.

On the basis of the data collected, physicians and nursing staff need to identify individual-specific problems and develop a care plan to address them.

The initial assessment process when the individual enters the health care organization determines what kind of care is required to meet the individual's primary needs. The reassessment process evaluates the individual's continuing needs, which change in response to care and treatment. Timely and accurate completion of assessments and reassessments by all caregiving disciplines can identify opportunities to improve an individual's overall status, thereby eliminating or reducing the need for restraint.

Accurate assessment allows a proactive evaluation of possible alternatives to restraint, if indicated during treatment.

Failure to complete assessments within the time frames specified by organization policies and procedures is a continuing problem in many health care organizations. Without proper and timely assessment, care planning and provision cannot be on target. The age and gender of care recipients—which are highly correlated with increased risk of restraint-related death or injury—must be considered. A description of specific assessment activities follows.

Assessment Activities

An individual's *physical status* often plays a central role in increasing risk for restraint or seclusion use. Physicians must ensure the inclusion of the following in physical status assessments.

Fall risk. Many physical conditions, in fact, increase an individual's risk for falls, which is one of the most frequent reasons restraint is used. Conditions include age; history of falls; irregular heartbeat; dizziness; vertigo; syncope; joint problems such as arthritis; muscle weakness; osteoporosis; paralysis or weakness due to cerebrovascular accidents; conditions that cause involuntary movements; unsteady gait or inability to control movements due to Parkinson's disease or other disorders; impaired vision, hearing, and speech (because the person may not be able to ask for help); lack of bowel and bladder control; dehydration; acute illnesses; casts, splints, prostheses, slings, and so forth; foot problems; poor posture or positioning; pain; and sensory impairment.

Nutritional status. Nutritional status should be part of an individual's physical assessment, whenever indicated. Nutrition can directly affect an individual's level of cognition, which in turn can directly affect the need for restraint. Timely identification and treatment by staff of nutritional issues, such as dehydration and malnutrition, can improve the cognitive status of patients.

Physical strength. Evaluation of each individual's physical strength is an important part of the physical assessment process. Through timely assessment and care planning, health care professionals can help ensure that physically weak individuals participate in muscle strengthening programs to improve sitting balance and eliminate the need for restraint.

Pain management needs. Physical assessment should include an assessment of the individual's pain management needs. Frequent attempts to get out of bed or out of restraints or to move to another location may be motivated by the individual's need for maximum comfort and relief of pain. Some individuals with cognitive impairments may exhibit agitated or aggressive behavior when experiencing pain but may be unable to express pain verbally. Health care team members should assess pain on admission and reassess on an ongoing basis.

Toileting needs. Attempts to get out of bed or restraints are often motivated by the individual's need to eliminate urine or stool. Hence, health care staff should ensure an accurate assessment of the care patient's toileting needs.

Medications. Initial and ongoing assessments must obtain information regarding medications the patient is receiving. Drugs can affect whether an individual is at increased risk of injury while in restraint or seclusion. Several classes of medications have been strongly associated with increased fall risk, which is highly correlated with restraint use. Multiple medications and combinations of medications can produce adverse reactions such as dizziness, increased agitation, sleeplessness, impaired balance, and other risk factors for restraint or seclusion use.

Thorough and accurate assessment of each individual's behavioral and cognitive status on admission and on a regular basis thereafter is key to reducing restraint or seclusion use. The depth of assessment should vary on the basis of the needs of the individuals served. For example, individuals who can communicate, listen, and solve problems are likely to be at lower risk for restraint or seclusion than individuals who are not able to communicate or listen or who have a history of aggressive episodes or increased motor agitation. The ehavioral/cognitive assessments of each should reflect this.

All patients with cognitive or sensory impairments, as well as those who are psychotic, severely emotionally disturbed, comatose, or ventilator dependent, must be assessed for pain. Like infants and children, cognitively impaired persons may signal pain or discomfort via behavioral factors.

In all health care organizations, a thorough assessment can identify individuals with cognitive issues. Inadequate perception of surroundings, mental disorientation, mood, decreased judgment, memory, attention span, confusion, and other cognitive issues can lead to the use of restraint. The initial assessment in long term care facilities might focus on whether the individual is confused or has a medical diagnosis such as Alzheimer's disease or dementia that increases the individual's risk for restraint use due to wandering, pacing, or fear of falls. Decline in cognitive skills, delirium, anxiety, anger, frustration, poor awareness of time, hallucinations, vivid dreams, and decreased ability to cope with stress place an individual at risk for falls and hence restraint use to reduce fall risk.

 Collaborate with other physicians and staff to develop and apply improved patient assessment processes. Physicians must be committed to reducing the use of restraint because of its risk for patient injury and death and must work with colleagues and organization leaders to devise proactive risk assessment procedures.

 Ensure the assessment and reassessment of all individuals in a timely and thorough manner, according to organization policies and procedures. The initial assessment

should be multidisciplinary and include physician participation. In collaboration with medical and nursing staff leaders, physicians must ensure that their patients receive thorough initial assessments and reassessments on a regular basis.

To reduce the risk of restraint-related injury or death, initial assessments must be performed in a timely manner for new admissions. In addition, reassessments documenting changes in patient conditions while in restraint must be performed and documented in a timely manner. The age and gender of patients—which are highly correlated with increased risk of restraint-related death or injury—must be considered. Any and all adverse or unusual effects of medications should be noted in the clinical record. The assessment activities should include those outlined earlier, as appropriate.

 Ensure the thorough identification of restraint alternatives. Ensure the participation and education of family members. Through the assessment process, physicians, nurses, and other team members can assist in identifying patients who may do well with measures other than physical restraints (see Sidebar 6-3). An in-depth nursing assessment and family interview provide the necessary background information. Education of family members can facilitate family cooperation in providing one-on-one supervision so that physical restraints do not need to be used. Family members can be taught therapeutic holding techniques that help to reduce the need for restraint or seclusion. Physicians can ensure that these alternatives are identified and that family participation is obtained.

 Ensure accurate assessment of each individual for the appropriateness of restraint use. Assessments must be customized for each individual. If an individual requires restraint, staff should identify the cause of the need for restraint and relate this to other assessment factors before communicating the need for restraint to the physician or others. For example, in acute care, where restraints are most often used to prevent falls and to maintain therapy, staff can evaluate patients who refuse to stay in bed for cognitive status, performance of activities of daily living, agitation, the presence of psychotropic drugs, and incidence of falls.[22] Restraint alternatives should be considered. A physician receiving a request for a restraint order must ask staff about the individual's assessment and how it indicated the appropriateness of restraint use.

System Solution 3: Care Planning and Provision

Near-Miss Example: Incomplete Communication

A woman is hospitalized in the ICU following a motor vehicle accident. With multiple broken bones and closed-head trauma, she requires multiple IV lines, a foley catheter, a cardiac monitor, and artificial ventilation. She also experienced severe seizures while being treated in the ED. The attending physician orders that both of her hands be restrained at all times. The physician does not specify the duration of the order, nor does he conduct an initial in-person evaluation within the required time frame.

On day two of caring for this individual, the nursing staff notes that the woman has had no further seizures and currently is lying calmly in the bed. After completing several tasks, the bedside nurse needs to dispose of some equipment away from the bedside but still in the room. In an effort to save time, the nurse places both siderails in the raised position but does not restrain the woman's upper extremities. With her back to the woman and on the opposite side of the room, the nurse hears slight movement. Returning quickly to the bedside, she discovers that in a brief amount of time, the woman has pulled out her foley catheter with one hand and dislodged the IV lines with the other hand. The nurse is able to correct the situation promptly.

Medical and nursing leaders must ensure that care, treatment, and rehabilitation are planned and

appropriate to each individual's needs. Then, health care staff must provide the care and treatment planned. Effective care and treatment reduce the likelihood of restraint use and concomitant risk of death and injury. Communication to all caregivers of the care plan goals and the approaches to those goals must be effective. Involvement and education of the individual and his or her family about goals and approaches help to reduce the likelihood of adverse events.

When restraint or seclusion is used for behavioral reasons or acute medical and surgical care reasons, individual orders provided by physicians and other appropriate health care staff guide their initial and continuing use and their discontinuation.* Individual orders provide the framework for ensuring clinical justification of restraint or seclusion use and for protecting the rights, dignity, and well-being of the care recipient. Individual orders must be consistent with organization policy and procedures and in accordance with state law.

According to Joint Commission requirements for hospitals and behavioral health care organizations, the LIP orders the use of restraint or seclusion. The LIP, a LIP designee, or another LIP must be primarily responsible for the patient's ongoing care.

The Joint Commission does not require a practitioner to have specific privileges to order restraint or seclusion; rather, this privilege is implied for all LIPs who have the appropriate competency.

The latest JCAHO provisions regarding delegation of restraint orders and evaluations by physicians and other LIPs in hospitals appear as Sidebar 6-5, page 116.

According to the *behavioral use standards,* a qualified staff member must notify and obtain an order (verbal or written) from the LIP as soon as possible,

---

* Clinical protocols can also be used to guide restraint or seclusion use for acute medical and surgical care reasons in acute medical and surgical hospitals and ambulatory settings.

Sidebar 6-5. Delegation of Restraint Orders and Evaluations in Hospitals

Effective July 1, 2002, LIPs in hospitals can delegate the writing of restraint or seclusion orders and/or the in-person evaluation of patients in restraint or seclusion to physician assistants and advanced practice nurses, if permitted by law and by the hospital.

When such delegation is permitted, the safety and quality of patient care are protected by

- the medical staff's responsibility for the quality of services provided by LIPs, including services provided through individuals to whom those LIPs delegate tasks;
- required supervision of physician assistants and advance practice nurses by LIPs; and
- requirements stating that all repeated or prolonged use of restraint or seclusion be reviewed by clinical leadership.

Source: Licensed independent practitioners may delegate restraint orders and evaluations in hospitals. *Jt Comm Persp* 22(5):6, May 2002.

but no longer than *1 hour* after the initiation of restraint or seclusion. The qualified staff member must also consult with the LIP about the individual's physical and psychological condition. At this point, the LIP also determines whether restraint or seclusion should be continued, supplies staff with guidance in identifying ways to help the individual regain control so that restraint or seclusion may be discontinued, and supplies an order.

According to the *acute medical and surgical use standards* for hospitals, an LIP must be notified within *12 hours* of the initiation of restraint, and a verbal order must be obtained from that practitioner and entered into the individual's clinical record. If the initiation of restraint is based on a significant change in the individual's condition, the registered nurse must immediately notify the LIP. A written order, based on an examination of the individual by an LIP, must be entered in the individual's clinical record within 24 hours of restraint initiation. If restraint use continues to be clinically justified, an LIP can authorize continued use of restraint beyond the first 24 hours by renewing the original order or issuing a new order. The renewal or new order, issued no less frequently than once each calendar day, is based on an examination of the individual by the LIP.

Prevention Strategy *Collaborate with other physicians and organization leaders to develop and apply high-quality restraint use policies and protocols.* When restraint is necessary, organization leaders must ensure physicians and all health care staff that patient safety will not be compromised. The development and implementation of safe restraint use policies and protocols require the full participation of physicians.

Prevention Strategy *Provide proper orders for restraint use.* Physicians and other LIPs need to be properly knowledgeable about the theory of physical restraint use and the need to limit use to a specific short duration. They also must know how to direct staff to use restraints through the orders the physicians provide. Each order needs to be specific about the type of device to be used and the reason for the device's use. Orders may be given to clinical staff only after all reasonable alternatives have been tried and failed and after documentation of attempts and failures appears in the clinical record.

Acceptable individual orders include at least the following elements:

- The start and end times and dates for restraint or seclusion;
- The type of restraint (if applicable);
- The signature of the LIP who gave the order;
- The signature of the individual who accepted the verbal order; and
- Review time frames, as defined by the organization.

Some organizations use a brightly colored peel-off note containing similar information to alert staff to reevaluate or rewrite an order. A sample order appears as Figure 6-2, page 118.

 Ensure appropriate time limits for restraint orders. Often physicians or other LIPs write "restrain as needed" or use physical restraint "PRN" (as needed). Joint Commission standards and laws in most states prohibit nursing staff from following such orders. The order needs to be time limited.

Joint Commission requirements are explicit about time limitations for restraint or seclusion use. When restraint or seclusion is used for *acute medical and surgical care reasons* by hospitals, individual orders cannot exceed 24 hours. When restraint or seclusion is used for *behavioral reasons* for hospitals or behavioral health care organizations, written and verbal orders for initial and continuing use must be time limited. Specific requirements are as follows:
- Verbal and written orders for restraint and seclusion are limited to
  - 4 hours for individuals ages 18 and older;
  - 2 hours for children and adolescents ages 9 to 17; and
  - 1 hour for children under age 9.
- No standing orders or PRN orders are permitted.

If restraint or seclusion needs to continue beyond the expiration of the time-limited order, the LIP primarily responsible for the individual's ongoing care, his or her LIP designee, or another LIP must provide a new order for restraint or seclusion.

Time-limited orders do not mean that restraint or seclusion must be applied for the entire length of time for which the order is written. JCAHO standards encourage the discontinuation of restraint or seclusion as soon as the individual meets the behavior criteria for its discontinuation. Physicians play a leadership role in multidisciplinary teams charged with the responsibility for defining this criterion in organization policies and procedures.

In instances in which restraint or seclusion is terminated before the time-limited order expires, the original order can be used to reapply the restraint or seclusion within the original time limit if the individual is again at imminent risk of physical harm to self or others and if nonphysical interventions are not effective. However, the LIP who is primarily responsible for the individual's ongoing care, his or her LIP designee, or another LIP must provide a new order for restraint or seclusion when the original order expires. Staff of hospitals subject to CMS rules should ensure compliance with the CMS regulation that states that a new order should be obtained even if the original order has not expired.

 Provide proper orders when restraint is used according to clinical protocols. Clinical protocols can be used to guide restraint or seclusion use for acute medical/surgical care reasons in acute medical and surgical hospitals and ambulatory care settings. Such protocols are not allowed under the new behavioral health care restraint and seclusion standards when restraint or seclusion is used for behavioral reasons on individuals with emotional or behavioral disorders.

A clinical protocol should place restraint in the context of a larger series of clinical care processes used for specific nonbehavioral health conditions and individuals. Restraint is not a clinical care treatment option. Restraint represents the failure of all other clinical care options and alternatives. The Joint Commission permits the use of clinical protocols that include restraint usage when the clinical protocol
- is focused on the clinical care of individuals (for example, individuals on ventilators, those with central lines) and represents a full continuum of use of alternatives prior to implementing the use of restraints;
- is approved by the medical staff when the organization has an organized medical staff or by the medical director in the absence of an organized medical staff;

Sample Restraint Order

Expires 24 hours after start time

Start date/time _____ and end date/time _____

The following assessment must be completed every calendar day and signed by a licensed independent practitioner (physician).

THE REASON FOR THE RESTRAINTS: Patient confused or otherwise unable to follow instructions and one or more of the following:

☐ Patient persists in efforts to disconnect medical equipment

☐ Patient thrashing in a manner and setting that could result in injury

☐ Patient picking at surgical/wound dressings in a manner that could compromise healing

☐ Patient exhibiting aggressive or violent behavior, potential for injury to the patient or other persons

☐ Other (specify) _____
_____

TYPE OF RESTRAINT

☐ Posey vest
☐ Soft limb
☐ Mittens
☐ Leather
☐ Elbow

ALTERNATIVES TO RESTRAINTS ATTEMPTED

☐ Sitter provided
☐ Verbal instructions
☐ Family member unable to stay with patient or provide sitters
☐ Modify environment
☐ Other (specify): _____
_____

Physician: _____ Date: _____

Keep this order sheet in front of current physician orders

Figure 6-2. This restraint order, developed by an acute care facility, indicates start and end dates and times, the reason for restraint use, the type of restraint, and alternatives attempted prior to restraint use. Note that the specified duration of restraint use (24 hours) applies only to use of restraint for acute medical and surgical care reasons.
Source: Sacred Heart Health System, Pensacola, FL. Used with permission.

- is ordered in writing by the LIP, to be implemented for each specific individual;
- contains specific criteria for determining when restraint is needed as part of the care (for example, sedation, confusion, self-extubation);
- identifies possible alternatives;
- is backed up with staff education and competence assessment for those who will use the protocol; and
- is consistent with organization policy.

The only acceptable protocol would be a clinical protocol that includes the use of restraints when all other treatment options and alternatives have failed. To use the protocol, there must be documented evidence that all other treatment options and alternatives have been attempted and have failed. A restraint protocol that describes solely when a restraint is used and is not part of the individual's clinical care is *not* considered a clinical protocol and does not meet Joint Commission standards. When restraint is initiated based on an approved protocol, its use must be authorized by an individual order.

The acute medical and surgical care standard for hospitals recognizes that during the treatment of certain specific conditions, such as posttraumatic brain injury, or the use of certain specific clinical procedures, such as intubation, restraint may often be necessary in order to prevent significant harm to the individual. Clinical protocols for the use of restraint may be established for specified conditions or procedures, based upon the frequent presentation of those conditions or procedures of behavior by individuals that seriously endangers the individual or seriously compromises the effectiveness of the procedure. Clinical protocols include

- guidelines for assessing the individual;
- criteria for applying restraint;
- criteria for monitoring the individual and reassessing the need for restraint; and
- criteria for terminating restraint.

Criteria for use of restraint that are included in such a protocol must reflect the organization's policies and procedures on the appropriate and safe use of restraint and must be approved by the medical staff, nursing leadership, and others, when appropriate, as specified by organization policy. Authorized staff can initiate, maintain, and terminate restraint based on these criteria, the individual's need, and appropriate justification. Staff must obtain an order for the clinical protocol's use, but if restraint is part of the protocol, staff do not have to obtain a separate order for restraint. However, staff must be trained and competent in use of the clinical protocol. For a sample clinical protocol used in acute care settings, see Figure 6-3, pages 120–121.

Prevention Strategy ***Evaluate the individual in restraint or seclusion.*** Physicians and other LIPs must evaluate the individual in restraint or seclusion in a face-to-face manner, except in those instances outlined in Sidebar 6-5. The LIP, his or her LIP designee, or another LIP might be the person primarily responsible for the individual's ongoing care.

During the in-person evaluation, the LIP works with the individual and staff to identify ways to help the individual regain control, makes any necessary revisions to the individual's treatment plan, and, if necessary, provides a new written order.

The time frame for the initial in-person evaluation is as follows:
- Within 1 hours of the initiation of restraint or seclusion for individuals ages 18 are older; and
- Within 2 hours of initiation for children and adolescents ages 17 and under.

If the individual is no longer in restraint or seclusion when the original order expires, the LIP conducts an in-person evaluation of the individual within 24 hours of the initiation of restraint or seclusion. A telemedicine link does not fulfill the in-person requirement for the evaluation by the LIP of the individual in restraint or seclusion.

Clinical Protocol for Restraint Use Related to Acute Medical and Surgical Care

An *intubated patient* may include a patient needing assistance with airway management via an endotracheal tube or tracheostomy.

A patient with *essential lines* or tubes necessary for medical treatment or life sustenance.

This protocol can be implemented by a competent registered nurse (RN) when the indicators are present and appropriate alternatives attempted.

A. **Criteria** - when the intubated patient or patient with essential lines or tubes demonstrates any of the following:
   1. Interference with medical devices, tubes, dressings.
   2. Unsteady gait; attempts to get up without assistance.
   3. Harmful to self.
   4. Severe agitation.
   5. Due to cognitive impairment, unable to follow commands or participate in plan of care.

B. **Alternatives** - attempt to use the following appropriate alternatives:
   1. Increase frequency of nursing rounds.
   2. Have the patients' family, significant other, and/or friends stay with the patient.
   3. Cover IV sites with fabric such as surginet.
   4. Cover PEG tube with an abdominal binder.
   5. Collaborate with the physician to:
      • Discontinue all tubes when medically possible.
      • Request tube feeding be changed to bolus when medically possible.
   6. Offer toileting at least q2h and as needed when restless and assure the bowel program has been effective.
   7. Ensure frequently needed items (i.e., urinal, phone, water, etc.) are located on unaffected side of cerebrovascular patient.

C. **Implementation** - if the above alternatives are ineffective, then the restraint protocol will be implemented by a qualified RN, based on an order from a licensed independent practitioner:
   1. Assessment of need will be evaluated each shift.
   2. An attempt to use an alternative to restraints will be assessed at least daily.
   3. Restraint protocol may be reinstated if the attempt to use alternatives is unsuccessful.
   4. Alternatives to restraints will be discussed weekly at interdisciplinary team meetings to determine if the need continues to be present and to explore additional alternatives.
   5. Any patient that does not meet protocol criteria will need a physician's order for restraints per hospital policy.

D. **Monitoring** - Monitoring patients as per Patient Restraints Policy.

E. **Documentation**

   Restraint Initiation Assessment
   • Reason for implementation of restraint.
   • Less restrictive alternatives attempted.
   • Education and patient/family responses.

   Restraint Observation Record
   • Assessment of continued need.
   • At least daily, attempt to remove restraint and record outcome.

F. **Termination** - when an alternative is available and/or the patient's behavior demonstrates no risk to him/herself or others, the restraint will be removed. The following criteria may be used:
   1. Improved mental status.
   2. No interferences with medical devices, tubes, dressings.
   3. Medical devices, tubes, dressings removed.
   4. Follows verbal commands.

(continued)

Figure 6-3. Developed by an acute care organization, this protocol covers use of restraint for an intubated patient or a patient with essential lines or tubes.

Clinical Protocol for Restraint Use Related to Acute Medical and Surgical Care (continued)

I. Clinical Justification for Restraints (Complete Section A for all patients) (Check all that apply.)

A. Behavior Necessitating Use of Restraint

☐ Interference with medical devices, tubes, dressings
☐ Unsteady gait; attempts to get up without assistance
☐ Harmful to self
☐ Severe agitation
☐ Due to cognitive impairment is unable to follow commands or participate in plan of care

COMPLETE SECTION B OR C AS APPROPRIATE

B. Behavior That Meets Criteria for Clinical Protocol for Intubated Patient or Patient with Essential Lines or Tubes

☐ Patient needs assistance with airway management via endotracheal tube or tracheostomy
☐ Patient needs lines or tubes for medical treatment for life sustenance

Confusion identified as an underlying component of the patient's medical condition:

☐ Organic Brain Syndrome
☐ Head Injury
☐ CVA
☐ Encephalopathy
☐ Other _____
AND MUST EXHIBIT AT LEAST ONE OF THE BEHAVIORS IN SECTION A

C. Patient Exhibits Behavior Necessitating Use of Restraint But Does Not Meet Criteria for Restraint Protocol

☐ If the initiation of restraint is based on a significant change in the patient's condition, notify the physician immediately and obtain order for restraint
☐ For Class I, II, or III, obtain physician order for restraint within 12 hours of restraint application
☐ For Class IV, obtain physician order for restraint within 1 hour of restraint application

II. Less Restrictive Alternatives to Restraints Attempted but Unsuccessful

☐ Increased frequency of nursing rounds
☐ Family/sitter present
☐ Cover IV sites, PEG, etc.
☐ Toileting at least q 2 hours
☐ Other _____

III. Education

☐ Family notified, name/relationship
☐ Notified by _____
☐ Comments _____
☐ Copy of restraint guidelines for patients and families given to and reviewed with patient/family
☐ Unable to educate due to _____

IV. RN Assessment

I have reviewed the data and assessed needs for restraint application

Date _____ Time _____ RN, Signature _____

CMS's requirements for hospitals participating in the Medicare and Medicaid programs are more stringent in this area. Effective August 1999, a physician or qualified LIP, as determined by each state, must evaluate an individual face-to-face within *one hour* of the initiation of restraint or seclusion use. The new CMS requirement has been very controversial in the health care community. CMS designed this "one-hour rule" to ensure that the restraint or seclusion is warranted and properly applied.[23] Organizations subject to Medicare Conditions of Participation must meet CMS's one-hour rule in order to comply with Joint Commission as well as CMS requirements because the Joint Commission requires organizations to comply with federal and state requirements.

Prevention Strategy *Reevaluate the individual in restraint or seclusion.* Physicians and LIPs must reevaluate individuals in restraint or seclusion in both hospitals and behavioral health care organizations.

Reevaluation of the individual takes place every
- 4 hours for adults ages 18 and older,
- 2 hours for children and adolescents ages 9 to 17, and
- 1 hour for children under age 9.

The physician or LIP who is primarily responsible for the individual's ongoing care, the LIP designee, another LIP, or an individual who meets the training and competence requirements to perform evaluations and reevaluations and who has been authorized by the organization to perform this function must perform the reevaluation.

New to this standard reference above is the requirement that an LIP conduct an in-person reevaluation at least every
- 8 hours for individuals ages 18 years and older; and
- 4 hours for individuals ages 17 and younger.

After the reevaluation is conducted, the LIP, his or her LIP designee, or another LIP must provide a written or verbal order if the restraint or seclusion is to be continued. In conjunction with the reevaluation, the LIP, qualified registered nurse, or other qualified, authorized staff member must reevaluate the efficacy of the individual's treatment plan and work with the individual to identify ways to help him or her regain control.

If the person conducting the reevaluation is not the LIP with primary responsibility for the individual's ongoing care, and if restraint or seclusion is to be continued, he or she must notify the LIP with primary responsibility for the individual's status.

System Solution 4: Observation and Monitoring

Sentinel Event Example: Inadequate Monitoring

A man receiving care in a behavioral health care facility experiences severe delirium, tremors, and hallucinations and begins to exhibit difficult and dangerous behavior. While notifying the man's physician and arranging to transfer the man to an appropriate acute care setting, staff are concerned about his safety and the safety of those around him. They try a variety of alternatives to the use of restraint, but each alternative is unsuccessful. While awaiting a return call from the man's physician, the staff place him in four-point restraint in the only area not currently occupied—a private room far from the nursing station. Because staffing is short that evening, no staff member is available to remain with the man, as specified in organization policies and procedures. Medical staff worked closely with an interdisciplinary restraint use team to develop observation protocols to assure safe restraint use. The charge nurse intends to return every five minutes for observations, as outlined in organization protocol when continuous observation is not possible. However, other critical situations develop, and the nurse does not return for almost one hour. At that time, the nurse finds the man unresponsive, having suffered a heart attack. He also has huge welts on all four extremities.

To prevent injury, individuals in restraints must be adequately monitored. If a restraint is used for too long, and if the individual is unable to move, health problems can occur, including pressure ulcers, nerve damage, and incontinence.[4] Psychological and physical decline can also occur, as illustrated in this example. Continuous observation of individuals in restraint can effectively reduce restraint-related deaths and injuries. Properly trained ancillary or volunteer staff, such as sitters, can be used to provide this one-on-one observation.

Organization leaders, including medical staff leaders, must ensure thorough monitoring policies and procedures, including proper documentation of observation, and physicians must be advised of the existence of such policies and procedures prior to admitting patients. Policies and procedures should address how frequently individuals in restraints should be observed. Requirements vary from program to program; one organization policy may not serve the needs of all programs. Organizations must be certain that their policies provide enough detail regarding observation procedures. All staff working in organizations with multiple programs and providing care in multiple settings should be competent with all policies and procedures.

Prevention Strategy *Ensure the observation of individuals receiving care.* One of the most effective methods of preventing the need for restraint is frequent observation and supervision of patients by nursing staff. Physicians can require this for patients in their care and make inquiries regarding how frequently observation occurs. Frequent monitoring of cognitively impaired individuals can alert staff members to early signs of restlessness or agitation, which may signal an increase in pain or discomfort that can be addressed before restraints or alternatives are necessary. High-risk individuals can be located close to nurses' areas to allow regular observation. Staff can identify individuals who are incontinent or who urinate frequently and place them on prompted voiding

schedules that allow for them to empty their bladders at least every two hours.

Concluding Comments

Using physical restraints is dangerous. Physicians can reduce the likelihood of restraint-related deaths or injuries by using alternatives to restraint whenever possible, ensuring proper education and training regarding alternatives, ensuring proper assessment, and ensuring timely and regular observation and monitoring of individuals in restraint. When restraint is needed, physicians can reduce the likelihood of restraint-related deaths or injuries by issuing proper, time-limited restraint orders and by evaluating and reevaluating individuals in restraint.

REFERENCES

1. Joint Commission on Accreditation of Healthcare Organizations: *Reducing Restraint Use in the Acute Care Environment.* Oakbrook Terrace, IL, 1998, p iv.
2. Joint Commission on Accreditation of Healthcare Organization: *Lexikon: Dictionary of Health Care Terms, Organizations, and Acronyms,* 2nd ed. Oakbrook Terrace, IL, 1998.
3. Food and Drug Administration: Safe use of physical restraint devices. *FDA Backgrounder,* Jul 1992. Web site: www.fda.gov/opacom/bacgrounders/safeuse.html.
4. Weiss EM: A nationwide pattern of death. *The Hartford Courant* 11 Oct 1998.
5. Joint Commission statistics provide insight into causes of sentinel events. *Jt Comm Persp* 22:3–5, Aug 2002.
6. Joint Commission: Preventing restraint deaths. *Sentinel Event Alert* Issue 8, 18 Nov 1998.
7. Frank C, Hodgetts G, Puxty J: Safety and efficacy of physical restraints for the elderly. *Can Fam Physician* 42:2402–9, Dec 1996.
8. Strumpf NE, Evans LK: Alternatives to physical restraints. *J Ger Nurs* 18(11):4, 1992.
9. Evans LK, Strumpf NE, Williams C: Redefining a standard of care for frail older people: Alternatives to routine physical restraint. In Katz P, Kane R, Mezey R (eds): *Advances in Long Term Care.* New York: Springer, 1991, pp 81–108.
10. Evans LK, Strumpf NE: Myths about elder restraint. Image: *J of Nurs Scholarship* 22(2):124–8, Summer 1990.
11. Sullivan-Marx EM: Physical and chemical restraints: Meeting the challenge. *Dimensions of Crit Care Nurs* 13:58–9, Mar/Apr 1994.
12. Tinetti M, Liu W, Ginter S: Mechanical restraint use and fall-related injuries among residents of skilled nursing facilities. *Ann Intern Med* 116(5):369–74, 1992.

13. Fletcher K: Use of restraints in the elderly. *AACN Clinical Issues* 7:611–20, Nov 1996.

14. Owens MF: Patient restraints: Protection for whom? *JONA's Healthcare Law, Ethics, and Reg* :59–65, Jun 2000.

15. Evans LK, Strumpf WE: Tying down the elderly. *J Am Geriatr Soc* 37(1):65–74, 1989.

16. Rubin BS, Dube AH, Mitchell EK: Asphyxial deaths due to physical restraint. *Arch Fam Med* 2:405–8, Apr 1993.

17. Strumpf NE, Evans LK: The ethical problems of prolonged physical restraint. *J Ger Nurs* 17:27–30, Feb 1991.

18. DiFabio S: Nurses' reactions to restraining patients. *Am J Nurs* 81:973–5, May 1981.

19. Scherer YK, et al: The nursing dilemma of restraints. *J Ger Nurs* 17:14–7, Feb 1991.

20. McHutchion E, Morse J: Releasing restraints: A nursing dilemma. *J Gerontological Nurs* 15(2):16–21, 1989.

21. Joint Commission on Accreditation of Healthcare Organizations: *Restraint and Seclusion: Complying with Joint Commission Standards.* Oakbrook Terrace, IL, 2002.

22. Werner P, et al: Individualized care alternatives used in the process of removing physical restraints in the nursing home. *J Am Geriatr Soc* 42:321–5, Mar 1994.

23. Albert T: Court backs rapid evaluation of patients in restraints. *Am Medical News,* 16 Oct 2000.

PROTECTING PATIENTS FROM SUICIDE

Hospitals and other 24-hour facilities are places for quality treatment and care. They are meant to be safe. How could suicide occur in such settings?

Cause for Concern

Every 18 minutes, one American commits suicide. Now the eleventh leading cause of death in the United States (the third for young persons), more than 30,000 people take their lives each year. Another approximately 730,000 attempt it, resulting in an estimated 5 million suicide survivors in the United States.[1] Approximately 2% to 6% of suicides are by individuals receiving treatment from health care professionals in hospital settings.[2] Suicidal behaviors are far more common among individuals receiving health care services than in the population at large. Approximately 12 persons per 100,000 commit suicide in the general population; in hospital settings, the rates range from 40 to 350 per 100,000 inpatients.[3] Studies indicate that of those persons committing a suicide, 50% saw physicians in the weeks prior to completing the act.[4]

Having suicidal thoughts or attempts is the most common reason for psychiatric inpatient admission. Reports indicate that between 60% and 75% of child, adolescent, and adult patients and 40% to 55% of geriatric patients are admitted to inpatient units with concerns of self-harm.[5] A considerable amount of research exists on the occurrence of suicide in hospital settings. Two researchers found that approximately one-third of inpatients who

commit suicide do so while on an authorized passes from health care facilities, another third after eloping from units, and the final third while within units. [3,6] Hanging is the most frequent suicide method on units, followed by jumping from a window or rooftop. Firearms are the most common method used outside units. Inpatient suicide most frequently occurs in bathrooms, followed by individuals' rooms.[3,7,8] High-risk periods are times of transition for an individual, including shortly after admission and just prior to or following discharge.[6,7]

Suicide has been the number-one type of sentinel event reviewed by the Joint Commission since implementation of the sentinel event policy in 1995. Of the more than 1,600 sentinel events reviewed from January 1995 through May 2002, nearly 281 (17.1%) were inpatient suicides.[9] Most of these suicides occurred in psychiatric hospitals and psychiatric units of general hospitals and to a lesser degree in medical/surgical units of acute general hospitals.[10] Some occurred in residential care facilities. In the vast majority of these cases, the method of suicide chosen by the individual was hanging in a bathroom, bedroom, or closet. In about 20% of the cases, individuals jumped to their death from a roof or out a window.

The Physician's Role

Physicians in all care settings play a primary role in assessing patients for suicide risk. Psychiatrists are normally assumed to be the type of physician most likely to evaluate suicidal patients. This certainly is true in hospital and behavioral heath care facilities.

However, as noted by one suicide risk advisory committee, "Non-psychiatric physicians, in their own practices, are treating an increasing number of depressed patients often with anti-depressant drugs. This implies an increasing need for sophistication in identifying patients at risk of killing themselves."[11] All physicians need to be aware of suicide risk factors and, while treating the patient as a whole, look for risk signs.

Physicians also have a responsibility to work with medical staff leaders to ensure that the facilities into which their patients are admitted are safe environments of care.

Common Systems Failures

Organizations that experienced inpatient suicides reviewed by the Joint Commission identified the following issues as root causes[10]:

- The environment of care, such as the presence of nonbreakaway bars, rods, or safety rails; lack of testing of breakaway hardware; and inadequate security;
- Patient assessment methods, such as incomplete suicide risk assessment at intake, absent or incomplete reassessment, and incomplete examination of the individual (for example, failure to identify contraband);
- Staff-related factors, such as insufficient orientation or training, incomplete competency review or credentialing, and inadequate staffing levels;
- Information-related factors, such as incomplete communication among caregivers and information being unavailable when needed; and
- Care planning, such as assignment of the patient to an inappropriate unit or location, and care provision, such as incomplete or infrequent observation.

The organizations reporting suicides cited the following as root causes or system failures[9]:
- The physical environment (89%);
- Inadequate assessment (75%);
- Insufficient staff orientation and training (62%);
- Communication failure (38%); and
- The lack of vital clinical information (29%).

Figure 7-1, page 127, provides the details. Physicians play a key role in the identification, assessment, and care of potentially suicidal individuals. A closer look at key system failures and prevention strategies follows.

System Solution 1: Assessment or Reassessment

Sentinel Event Example 1: Inadequate Assessment

A man is admitted to the surgical unit of a hospital for evaluation and observation the night prior to his planned surgery to remove a cancerous lung tumor. He has had a biopsy, and the diagnosis and plan are clear. The man's wife had called the oncologist's office earlier the same day to report symptoms of what the oncologist suspects is depression. The hospital's inpatient assessment process does not include a screen to identify patients at risk of suicide.

Early that evening, the man kisses his wife "good night" and tells her he will see her in the morning. Later that evening, he gets himself ready for bed and turns off his light. At 10:30 PM, the nurse hears a very loud crash coming from the man's room. She hurries into the room, notes that the window has been shattered and that the man is no longer in the room. She runs to the window and sees the patient six stories below, lying facedown. Security personnel, nurses arriving for the night shift, and visitors have responded and are summoning help. The man is transported to the ED, where he is pronounced dead.

Sentinel Event Example 2*: Inadequate Assessment

---

*   This example appears courtesy of Risk Management Foundation: RMF guidelines for identification, assessment, and treatment planning for suicidality. *Forum* 20:4–5, Fall 2000. Used with the permission of the Risk Management Foundation of the Harvard Medical Institutions.

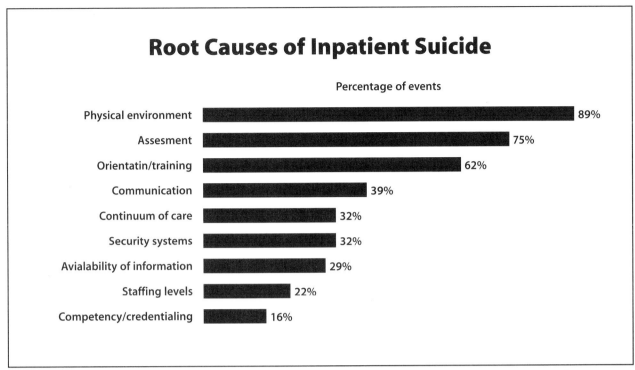

Figure 7-1. This chart illustrates the percentage of causes at the root of inpatient suicides reviewed by the Joint Commission between January 1995 and May 2002.

A 27-year-old patient was admitted to a psychiatric facility with a diagnosis of severe depression with suicidal ideation (thoughts of suicide). Several weeks later, the patient was given his first overnight pass to go home with his mother. The patient's antidepressant medication was not mentioned in the pass order written by the physician, and the patient went home without it. His mother called the next morning to say that her son was anxious and did not sleep. She was instructed to bring him back to the hospital. While stopped at a bridge toll booth en route, the patient left his mother's car and jumped off the bridge to his death.

These examples illustrate the danger of inadequate assessment. As mentioned earlier, inadequate assessment is the most frequently identified root cause of inpatient suicide. The purpose of assessment is to obtain appropriate and necessary information about each patient at times of entry into or transition within a health care setting or service. The information is used to match an individual's need with the appropriate setting, care level, and

intervention. The purpose of suicide assessment is to identify individuals at increased risk for suicide and to obtain clinical information relevant to their treatment planning. Periodic reassessment assures ongoing monitoring of suicide risk over time. The Joint Commission requires organizations to have an assessment procedure for the early detection of problems that are life threatening.

An initial screening, based on demographic characteristics of the individual and clinical and psychological indicators, provides the information necessary to determine whether suicide assessment is warranted. Although suicide risk is commonly not considered with individuals who come into the acute care setting for medical or surgical reasons, the first example indicates that physicians and other care staff members must consider suicide risk with all patients.

Assessments of medical or surgical patients should consider each individual's perception of the disease and the plan of treatment. Cancer patients are often

Sidebar 7-1.
Suicide Risk Factors

- Previous suicide attempt
- History of depression or other mood disorders, including schizophrenia and bipolar disorder
- Victim of sexual abuse, particularly incest, domestic violence, or other assault
- Witness to a suicide
- Alcohol or substance abuse
- Recent loss (of significant other or job, for example)
- Unnecessary risk-taking or self-destructive behaviors
- Chronic or terminal illness or uncontrollable pain
- Sudden change in normal behavior or attitude
- Presence of a suicide plan and final arrangements
- Presence of firearms

A thorough and insightful assessment of the individual's psychological state prior to surgery may indicated that the person is unhappy, nervous, and perhaps depressed. Referral of such a patient to a professional in psychology or psychiatry prior to surgery on the basis of such an observation would at the very least improve the individual's level of comfort and might avert a more serious outcome, as in the example of the man with lung cancer. A thorough pre-overnight leave assessment of the young man described in the second example should have probed for increased suicidal ideation. The overnight-pass documentation itself should have provided detailed instructions to the young man's mother about medications required and warning signs of at-risk status to report to facility staff.

Physicians or other clinicians must determine whether the individual presents low, moderate, or high suicide risk. Many organizations have compiled lists of common clues, danger signs, or risk factors that indicate potentially suicidal individuals and the need to seek professional help for suicide assessment and intervention. Physicians should be able to identify patients who have multiple diagnoses or risk factors that, in combination, can increase the risk of suicide. A list of commonly cited suicide risk factors appears as Sidebar 7-1, left.

Physicians and the organizations with which they are affiliated must ensure that potentially at-risk patients are asked whether they have recently or in the past considered or attempted suicide. Reassessment is critical before patients leave the facility on home passes. Suicidal ideation as well as actual attempts are factors that significantly increase suicide risk and must be taken seriously.

Physicians often need to rely on a nursing screen and assessment of the potential "lethality" of all individuals who are admitted to the health care organization, particularly persons with depression. It is not unusual for an individual to be admitted to a psychiatric unit in the middle of the night. In

despondent. They may fear a slow and painful death, the strain on family members, and the sapping of family resources.

Hence, physicians should be encouraged to participate in the assessment process or, at the very least, ensure that the psychosocial portion of the assessment is thoroughly completed either by themselves or by nursing or other appropriate staff. As surgical nurses would generally attest, physical assessment is well addressed in initial and ongoing assessment. The patient is physically prepared for the procedure, his or her vital signs are appropriate to allow the procedure, the necessary IV lines have been started, and the sites have been marked to assure surgery of the correct side, site, or limb. As a counterpart, the psychosocial assessment should address the individual's understanding of the disease and answer such questions as Who does the individual live with? What are the patient's expectations of the planned surgery? What does the patient feel will be the impact on his or her life and that of the family?

many hospitals, particularly small rural hospitals, a psychiatrist may not be available. Many individuals attempt suicide within the first few hours in the organization.

A true assessment of the lethality of the individual's suicidal ideation or potential must be conducted. This can be accomplished only with adequate historical information and is most productive if the organization has established clinical criteria to determine the degree to which intent in the individual's threats would lead to an attempt. Criteria include the number of previous suicidal episodes, how they have been manifested, and what information can be obtained that would suggest that an individual might attempt suicide. The influence of illicit substances is extremely important as well.

Proper assessment involves routinely asking individuals about their recent and past suicidal thoughts, feelings, and plans. Asking the suicide ("S") question—"Have you ever had thoughts of killing yourself?"—is the direct way to ask the question to detect suicide risk. Yet the question is frequently an uncomfortable one for staff members and may go unasked during initial and ongoing assessments. Compounding this, patients may be reluctant without a prompt to raise thoughts and feelings about suicide because of their own discomfort about the subject. Possible "S" questions to ask during an initial assessment appear in Sidebar 7-2, right.

Paul Quinnett, PhD, and his colleagues at Greentree Behavioral Health in Spokane, Washington, suggest asking the "S" question while obtaining background and family history for mental illness, substance abuse, and depression and mood disorders. In their suicide risk reduction program for hospitals, they write, "The 'S' question can be asked as follows, 'Has anyone in your family been depressed or seen a psychiatrist or counselor? Has anyone ever threatened, made an attempt, or committed suicide?' This can then be followed by, 'Have you ever

---

Sidebar 7-2. Suicide Screening Questions for an Initial Assessment

The following questions represent a sampling of possible suicide screening questions:

- Have you had thoughts of death or of killing yourself? What were they?
- What did you think about doing to yourself?
- Are you currently thinking about killing yourself?
- What are your thoughts on how, when, and where you would do this?
- Have you attempted suicide in the past? What did you do?
- Has a close friend or anyone in the family committed suicide?
- Has anyone in the family ever been treated for depression or emotional illness?
- Have you tried to hurt yourself? If so, how?

---

experienced thoughts of death or suicide or have you ever heard voices telling you to kill yourself?'"[12] The only way not to ask the question, according to Quinnett, is by phrasing it in a manner such as, "You're not thinking about suicide, are you?" This increases the individual's anxiety and sets up a negative response.

"Clinicians tend to make assessment errors at two points in the continuum of care: the first is soon after the individual is admitted and the second is when the person is starting to look and act better, showing sudden signs of improvement," says one behavioral health care surveyor for the Joint Commission. "The new patient figures out how to commit suicide before the staff really gets a feel for him or her; the seemingly improved individual may be improved only because he or she has developed a suicide plan and medications have kicked in, providing the energy and focus to actually act on the plan," says the surveyor.[13]

One Joint Commission sentinel event specialist recommends that physicians and other clinicians treat sudden shifts of behavior as red flags that indicate the need for in-depth suicide assessment. These shifts are temporary and purposefully mislead clinical improvements.[13] The specialist suggests not leaving new patients alone, particularly those for whom little information is available on admission. The associate director of the Joint Commission's Division of Research recommends thorough assessment of the patient before any passes or outings are approved. "If the staff has any worries about the individual's safety, the person should not be allowed to leave the facility," says the associate director.[13]

 Collaborate with other physicians, medical staff leaders, and other health care staff to develop and implement a protocol for suicide risk assessment. A uniform, standardized approach to suicide risk assessment and documentation increases the likelihood that the right clinical questions will be asked and relevant information obtained.[5] "If an inpatient service uses a standardized assessment form, however, there should be a clear understanding that the form does not substitute for clinical judgment, and whatever uniform approach is used, adequate opportunity should be left for the clinician to make additional comments or observations," notes one author.[5] Physicians should be part of a multidisciplinary team that includes nurses, social workers, and other mental health professionals and is responsible for creating and implementing a suicide risk assessment protocol.

 Ensure that all admissions are screened for suicidal ideation. Physician should ensure that all patients admitted to psychiatric units of general hospitals and psychiatric hospitals are screened for suicidal ideation. All individuals should be asked the "S" question. Physicians and all staff should ask the individual about suicide as sensitively as possible, avoiding use of any words or statements that could seem judgmental. Research indicates that talking about

suicidal thoughts provides relief for the patient. Suicide-specific questions recommended by one organization for all clinicians who conduct psychiatric evaluations include the following[11]:

- Are suicidal thoughts/feelings present?
- What form does the patient's wish for suicide take?
- What does suicide mean to the patient?
- How far has the suicide planning process proceeded?
- Has the patient engaged in self-mutilating behaviors?
- Does the patient's mental state increase the potential for suicide?
- Are epidemiologic risk factors present?

 Be a good listener and ensure that you obtain complete information. Active listening is critical during the assessment process, as are complete answers. If necessary, the physician or other clinician patient should ask the patient to provide more information and give the person time to respond. Individuals who are experiencing psychological stress about treatment may need more prompting for complete answers and more time to respond. Communication with the patient's family may be helpful in identifying individuals at risk for suicide. Confidentiality should be considered and maintained.

 Ensure reassessment during high-risk times of transition. Because change is stressful for many patients, times of transition are high-risk periods for suicide in a 24-hour care setting. Hence, physicians and other health care leaders must ensure that staff reassess patients at these times. As mentioned earlier, the period shortly after an individual is admitted is a high-risk time. The individual may still have a viable suicide plan and the intent to implement it. In addition, suicide risk is especially high at the time of discharge. The transition from inpatient to outpatient care is often problematic because, for example, the individual may be anxious about returning to an unsheltered and nonsupportive environment.

Thorough reassessment prior to granting an individual a pass or increased privileges is critical because of the high frequency of suicide while individuals are out on passes or authorized visits. The second example illustrates the importance of thorough reassessment at such a time and the need for thorough communication with the family regarding medications and at-risk behavior. Clinicians should assess what support systems are available to the individual on a pass. If support from family or friends is not available; if family will increase the individual's stress, anger, or other adverse emotions; or if the physician or another clinician has any worries about the individual's safety, the person should not be allowed to leave the facility. In addition, the patient should be reassessed on return from passes or other special privileges. The stress of visiting an unchanged home environment that may have precipitated the crisis, or negative interactions with others during the pass, can rekindle suicidal ideation. Also, passes may permit depressed individuals access to the means of completing suicide that are not available in health care settings. Passes may also permit access to illegal substances that could affect the individual's mood and hence suicidal intent. See Sidebar 7-3, right, for a summary of situations requiring suicide risk assessment and documentation.

System Solution 2: Environment of Care

Sentinel Event Example: Suicide

The police bring a 50-year-old man to a large urban hospital at 12:30 AM. The man had been in the town "lockup" since 7:00 PM, following an altercation with his girlfriend. While in police custody, the man had become progressively more despondent and had made statements suggesting that he wanted to commit suicide.

Following assessment in the ED by an emergency physician, the man is admitted to a 50-bed acute psychiatric unit for in-depth evaluation of suicide risk. Following an initial screen by nursing staff, a psychiatrist assesses the man and conducts an interview. The

---

Sidebar 7-3. Situations Requiring Suicide Risk Assessment and Documentation

- On admission;
- When the individual exhibits suicidal behavior or expresses suicidal thoughts;
- When a clinical or behavioral change occurs;
- Prior to granting increased privileges or a pass;
- When the individual returns from a pass; and
- Prior to discharge.

---

psychiatrist asks the man if he currently has or has had suicidal thoughts. Speaking with considerable anxiety, the man indicates that he had made threats in the police department so that he could get out of jail. He tells the psychiatrist that he is not contemplating suicide and that he does not have a suicide plan. The man signs an agreement that he will not hurt himself. The psychiatrist places him on a 20-minute observation schedule.

A mental health worker makes rounds about 25 minutes later. The worker finds the man sitting on the toilet, slumped forward, hanging from the water supply pipe of the toilet. The man had torn his T-shirt into strips of sufficient length to tie around his neck and around the flush mechanism on the toilet's water supply pipe. The worker calls a code, but resuscitative efforts are unsuccessful.

Environmental factors contributed to this man's suicide completion. A pipe was available for his use in hanging himself. Multiple environmental opportunities, beyond the obvious, present themselves to individuals inclined to carry out suicide. Physicians and other staff caring for individuals at risk for suicide should be aware of these hazards and help ensure their removal. The organization in this example might already have replaced shower curtain rods with breakaway rods and showerheads with beveled or breakaway shower heads, as recommended by experts. However, staff failed to identify other environmental hazards, such as the toilet's water supply pipe. Many toilets do not have fill tanks but have high-pressure-flush hardware from which an individual can hang him or herself. Some organizations have recognized this problem and have recessed the plumbing into the wall behind the toilet, leaving only a push button exposed. Disability grab bars present another hazard because individuals can wrap string, a belt, or an article of clothing around them to commit suicide. These bars can be designed with sloping attachments such that they could not be used to support an attempted hanging. Physicians must be familiar with the environments in which their patients receive care and must work with organization leaders to ensure a safe environment of care.

Prevention Strategy *Be knowledgeable about environmental hazards and advocate for their removal.* Physicians, along with nursing staff, need to be aware of areas and elements of the environment that represent opportunities for individuals intent on committing suicide. The removal of environmental hazards is particularly important for an individual who has clear signs of suicidal tendencies with significant lethality. Under such circumstances, frequent evaluation or even one-on-one observation should be implemented. Nevertheless, a general awareness of how individuals could carry out suicide is important for physicians and nurses to possess.

Because hanging is the most common method of inpatient suicide, a popular myth about hanging should be addressed. David M. Sine, consultant to the National Association of Psychiatric Health Systems, mentions that there is a widely pervasive misconception of what it takes to hang oneself in modern society. "Someone intent on suicide doesn't need to figure out a way to suspend his or her whole body weight. All they have to do is wrap something around their neck, attach it to something solid, and

lean forward, even from a kneeling position. It takes much less weight than many think," explains Sine.[14] Door hinges, doorknobs, nonbreakaway bathroom fixtures, exposed lighting fixtures, closet poles, metal hangers, and other potential environmental hazards should be removed, whenever possible. Physicians can help advocate for this. Sidebar 7-4, page 133, presents other recommendations regarding the environment of care. Understanding of the threats in the environment and completion of a thorough assessment of the individual's intent to commit suicide provide a critical opportunity for caregivers in psychiatric units and facilities to implement appropriate observation and control measures. Individuals who are at risk should be moved to areas where continuous observation can occur until lethality of suicidal tendencies has abated. Staffing should be adjusted to consider environmental hazards that cannot immediately be addressed. When substantive changes to the environment are not possible, close observation of the patient is the best strategy.

Prevention Strategy *Ensure that organization leaders examine the care environment for safety and security considerations.* Leaders are required to ensure the design of a safe, accessible, effective, and efficient environment of care that meets the needs of individuals served. A potentially suicidal individual presents significant challenges in this regard. Management plans must address safety and security, and such plans must be implemented. Organizations must meet the challenge of providing a safe environment of care while maintaining individual rights, such as the right to privacy, dignity, and a therapeutic environment. Physicians can be effective advocates for a safe environment and, as part of multidisciplinary teams, can provide important insights about suicide prevention.

System Solution 3: Orientation and Training

Sentinel Event Example: Inadequate Observation

An 80-year-old man in a long term care facility appears to be complying with his medication therapy.

Two times each day, a staff member delivers his medication dose to his room. However, he fakes swallowing his pills and moves them with his tongue into the space between the cheek and lower or upper gums (the "buccal gutter"). Once the staff member leaves his room, he removes the medications from his mouth and stores the pills in a hiding place in his clothes drawer. Eight days later, he takes all the medications at once, causing a fatal arrhythmia and death by overdose.

Staffing levels and the orientation and training of staff play a major role in an organization's effort to reduce suicide risk. In this example, training and appropriate observation of the patient are issues. Staff orientation and training are key to the proper assessment of suicidal risk and the prevention of suicide. Physicians knowledgeable about suicide risk can play an important role in working with medical, nursing, and other leaders to develop and implement an effective suicide assessment and prevention program.

At the completion of orientation, all staff members must demonstrate knowledge, skills, and competence sufficient to assume assigned responsibilities. Organization leaders must ensure that all staff with direct contact with patients receive education about the prevalence of suicide in health care settings. Too often, suicide "pacts" between patients and staff are taken as gospel that individuals will not attempt to harm themselves. Yet, all along, an individual may be continuing to prepare for suicide in subtle ways that may not be recognized by a caregiver whose training or observation skills are inadequate. All staff members administering medications need to be aware of the practice of placing medications into the buccal gutter, sometimes called "cheeking." Oral examination after a patient swallows medications may be a requisite for those who have been known to hide medications.

How can physicians affect staff orientation and training?

Sidebar 7-4. Environment of Care Recommendations

Although most experts agree that it is not possible to "suicide proof" any space, the following recommendations can remove the most obvious environmental hazards:

- Identify and remove or replace nonbreakaway hardware in bathing facilities.
- Assure that existing breakaway hardware has been appropriately weight tested.
- Redesign, retrofit, or introduce security measures (for example, locking mechanisms, patient monitors, and alarms).
- Keep the patient's personal laundry facilities closed and locked and implement systems to monitor individuals who need to do their laundry.
- Remove plastic liners from trash cans to prevent asphyxiation by packing the oropharynx or placing bags over the head.
- Shorten the nurse call pull cords in bathrooms so they cannot be used for strangulation.

 Collaborate with medical staff leaders and organization leaders to enhance staff education on suicide risk assessment and patient monitoring. Physicians can play a powerful advocacy role in ensuring that all staff receive thorough education regarding suicide risk assessment and the care of potentially suicidal patients. Orientation of new staff is crucial. No staff members should be allowed to work in care areas until they demonstrate a thorough understanding of all the aspects of assessment and care of the specific patient population. Following orientation, the competence of the caregiver in managing potentially suicidal individuals in crisis includes the following:

- Excellence in assessment skills to determine from the individual's level of agitation, despondency, and behavior that this is an individual in crisis.

Sometimes a calm and composed person has resolved to carry out a suicide.

- An understanding of the environment of care and of where the individual should be placed in the unit if not all the rooms have been made as free of hazards as possible.
- An understanding of the individual's medication needs and of when the individual should be medicated.

Competence must be assessed on a regular basis. Physicians can work with organization leaders to ensure that proper training and competence assessment processes are in place.

System Solution 4: Communication, Information Availability, and Care Planning

Incomplete communication among caregivers or the lack of vital information when needed can increase the risk of suicide. Inadequate observation can do likewise. The purpose of an interdisciplinary treatment planning process in all care settings is to ensure that all caregivers are aware of each patient's needs so that care interventions can be collaboratively implemented by caregivers from a variety of disciplines. Communication provides the foundation for this process. If some caregivers are not adequately informed of an individual's needs, sentinel events can ensue. Transmission of data and information must be timely, accurate, and complete among all health care professionals. Physicians and other health care staff must ensure that the patient's clinical record contains sufficient information to support clinical decisions. Past suicide attempts, triggers that may influence behaviors, and any recent changes that have occurred in the person's life must be identified by the treating physician and organization staff. The review of data related to admission to other organizations may play a key role in identifying a patient who is at risk for suicide. The accurate and timely sharing of this information among caregivers is crucial to providing the best care in the safest possible environment.

Following initial assessment of the potentially suicidal individual, the physician and organization staff should develop a care plan tailored to meet the individual's needs. As the individual receives care, suicide risk should be reassessed and the care plan revised as appropriate to treatment goals and results. Leaders must work with physicians to ensure that the care plan fully reflects the individual's assessment and reassessment findings and that the care plans varies by risk levels. Sidebar 7-5, page 135, describes risk categories used by many organizations. These risk levels should tie to specific treatment protocols that have been developed by the medical staff. For example, a high-risk individual would be placed on continuous observation. Level of risk categories, determined during an assessment, should correlate with level of care decisions, determined during the care planning process. In turn, level of care decisions should identify the specific suicide precaution level appropriate to each individual. Leaders must work with physicians to establish clear policies on monitoring levels and ensure that these are reflected in policies and procedure manuals and effectively communicated to all staff.

The care plan initiated by the physician must be understood and implemented by all members of the care team. The plan must address the patient's specific needs and the multidisciplinary interventions to meet such needs. If the care plan calls for observation, for example, the observation level must be delineated clearly so that none of the caregivers has questions about what such observation entails.

The treatment plan must address as a primary function the individual's safety. The plan provides the physician's basis for appropriate observation of the individual in the care setting and for participation in therapeutic activities. Revision of the plan may be required when changes are noted in the individual's condition or behavior. Physicians must ensure that all caregivers receive critical information regarding plan revision.

Care planning problems have been identified as one of the root causes of many of the suicides reviewed by the Joint Commission. Such problems include assignment of the individual to an inappropriate unit or location and placement of the suicidal individual in seclusion with restraints as standard operating procedure.

Physicians can implement proactive strategies to enhance care planning and communication and information transfer, thereby reducing suicide risk.

 Help ensure complete information transfer on admission. An organization's admission policies and procedures should minimize the occurrence of admission of individuals for whom medical and psychiatric histories are unavailable. When information on admission is insufficient, nursing and other staff cannot ensure the individual's safety. Physicians must provide appropriate clinical information on all patients admitted to health care organizations. The increased availability of electronic medical records facilitates this process.

 Document and communicate key assessment findings. Once the initial admission assessment has occurred, findings need to be thoroughly documented and properly communicated to all clinical staff. On occasion, staff may complete an assessment within the required time frame but then forget to include the material in the clinical record or communicate significant findings to appropriate colleagues. Documentation must occur within the required time frame, and the documents must be signed and validated by a physician. The information cannot be waiting on a transcription line somewhere. It has to be available to caregivers to aid in decision making. For example, if assessment findings indicate that an individual is at high risk for suicide, staff must be informed immediately in order to implement line-of-sight or even arm's length, one-to-one observation procedures.

Sidebar 7-5.
Suicide Risk Levels

- *Lowest risk:* Individual expresses no thoughts of death.
- *Low risk:* Individual expresses thoughts of death, but not by suicide.
- *Moderate risk:* Individual expresses suicidal thoughts without having considered the specific method.
- *High risk:* Individual expresses suicidal thoughts and has determined a specific plan.

Help ensure complete information transfer during provision of care. Thorough communication among the staff involved in the care of a potentially suicidal individual is a critical factor in reducing the risk of suicide. Information about changes in an individual's behavior, however small, may signal a trend and must be communicated to caregivers on the current and next shift. For example, if a person's behavior improves dramatically and the person starts cleaning his or her room, participating in groups sessions, and so forth, staff should document and communicate these behaviors from one shift to another. Behavior such as slowly giving away possessions to other patients or having family members take articles home can also be signs of renewed suicidal ideation. Documentation via written notes in the chart or verbal reports should prompt reassessment of the individual for the availability of a suicide plan. All high-risk thoughts, feelings, and behaviors exhibited or expressed by an individual must be clearly communicated to other caregivers.

Thorough information transfer must occur during all phases of care. Communication at the time of shift change is particularly important. The oncoming shift needs to be aware of issues related to specific aspects of each individual's care. Communication of changes to physicians who may not be on the unit at all times is critically important. Through initial and revised orders, physicians specify the interventions required to care for each individual. Lack of communication to all members of the team regarding patient changes can be devastating.

 Help ensure complete information transfer prior to discharge. Because discharge represents a transition for an individual—a high-risk time for suicide—the thorough transfer of information and thorough communication are particularly critical at this point. The individual and family or significant others should be informed by physicians, nurses, or other health care staff about what might increase the risk of the return of suicidal tendencies, such as discontinuation of medications and noncompliance with the treatment plan. They also should be informed about ongoing treatment needs, community resources, and how to access emergency services after discharge.

 Help ensure completion of all assessments prior to initiation of care planning. To ensure appropriate care, all disciplines' assessments, including the physician assessment, must be up to date and completed prior to the initiation of effective care planning.

Lead the care planning process and communicate care plan details to involved caregivers. Physicians generally direct the care planning and help to ensure adequate documentation of the interdisciplinary care plan and its dissemination to all disciplines and caregivers involved. Physicians should also communicate the tenets of the care plan to the patient. A patient needs to buy into the plan of care if satisfactory results are to be achieved and the risk of suicide reduced.

Help ensure implementation of the appropriate observation level. Implementation of the suicide precautions written by a physician or an other clinician specifying a level of surveillance of the

individual by nursing or assistive staff is critical. Precautions involve constant or intermittent observation or some gradation thereof. Physicians can enlist the assistance of nursing staff to ensure implementation of the appropriate observation level.

 Communicate the need to change an individual's observation level. Just as choosing the initial observation level requires considerable thought, so does increasing or decreasing the monitoring level. In some organizations, nurses, social workers, or others are allowed to implement a stricter, more protective monitoring level, and orders from a physician or other LIP are required for a decreased monitoring level. Evaluation and feedback from the observer team are critical to changing monitoring levels.

 Help ensure thorough implementation of observation policies and procedures. Leaders must ensure thorough implementation of observation procedures and monitor staff performance of such procedures.

Concluding Comments

Physicians, nurses, and other health care staff can proactively prevent patient suicides by working as a team to ensure adequate patient assessment and reassessment; a safe environment of care; proper orientation, training, and competence assessment; sufficient staffing; complete communication; accurate and timely information transfer; thorough care planning; and high-quality care provision.

REFERENCES

1. American Association of Suicidology (AAS): 1999 National Suicide Statistics and Facts. 17 Nov 2001. Web site: www.suicidology.org.
2. Busch KA, et al: Clinical features of inpatient suicide. *Psych Annals* 23(5):256–62, 1993.
3. Farberow NL: Guidelines to suicide prevention in the hospital. In Shneidman ES, Farberow NL, Litman RL (eds): *The Psychology of Suicide: A Clinician's Guide to Evaluation and Treatment.* Northvale, NJ: J. Aronson, 1994.

4. Blumenthal SJ: Suicide: A guide to risk factors, assessment, and treatment of suicidal patients. *Med Clin North Am* 72(4):937–71, 1988.

5. Jacobson G: The inpatient management of suicidality. In Jacobs DG (ed): *The Harvard Medical School Guide to Suicide Assessment and Intervention.* San Francisco: Jossey-Bass, 1999, p 38.

6. Litman RE: Suicide prevention in a treatment setting. *Suicide Life Threat Behav* 25(1):134–42, 1995.

7. Busch KA, Clark DC, Kravitz HM: Clinical features of inpatient suicide. *Psychiatr Annals* 23(5):256–62, 1993.

8. Cardell R, Horton-Deutsch SL: A model for assessment of inpatient suicide potential. *Arch Psychiatr Nurs* 8(6):366–72, 1994.

9. Joint Commission Resources: Statistics provide insight into causes of sentinel events. *Jt Comm Persp* 22:3–5, Aug 2002.

10. Joint Commission: Inpatient suicides: Recommendations for prevention. *Sentinel Event Alert* Issue 7, 6 Nov 1998.

11. Risk Management Foundation: RMF guidelines for identification, assessment, and treatment planning for suicidality. *Forum* 20:4–5, Fall 2000.

12. Cardell R, Quinnett P, Bratcher K: QPRT-H *Suicide Risk Management Inventory—Hospital Version.* Spokane, WA: Cardell, Quinnett, and Bratcher, 1999.

13. As quoted in Joint Commission: Asking the "suicide question": Assess thoroughly and often to reduce risk. *Jt Comm Benchmark* 1:1–3, Aug 1999.

14. Personal communication with David Sine, Jun 1999.

SELECTED RESOURCES

Joint Commission Books

Failure Mode and Effects Analysis in Health Care: Proactive Risk Reduction (2002)

Front Line of Defense: The Role of Nurses in Preventing Sentinel Events (2001)

Medication Use: A Systems Approach to Reducing Errors (1998)

Preventing Adverse Events in Behavioral Health Care: A Systems Approach to Sentinel Event (1999)

Preventing Medication Errors: Strategies for Pharmacist (2001)

Preventing Patient Suicide (2000)

Reducing Restraint Use in the Acute Care Environment (1998)

Restraint and Seclusion: Complying with Joint Commission Standards (2002)

Root Cause Analysis in Health Care: Tools and Techniques, Second Edition (2003)

Sentinel Events: Evaluating Cause and Planning Improvement (1998)

Storing and Securing Medications (1998)

Using Hospital Standards to Prevent Sentinel Events (2001)

What Every Hospital Should Know About Sentinel Events (2000)

Other Resources

This list includes selected classic and recent books, articles, presentations, and reports.

American Academy of Orthopaedic Surgeons: Advisory Statement: Wrong-site surgery. Web site: www.aaos.org/wordhtml/papers/advistmt/wrong.htm. American Academy of Orthopaedic Surgeons: Report of the task force on wrong-site surgery. Web site: www.aaos.org/wordhtml/meded/tasksite.htm.

American Academy of Orthopaedic Surgeons: Sign your site: Wrong site surgery. Web site: www3.aaos.org/wrong/viewscrp.cfm.

American Society of Health-System Pharmacists: Suggested definitions and relationships among medication misadventures, medication errors, adverse drug events, and adverse drug reactions. Web site: www.ashp.com/public/proad/mederror/draftdefin.html.

Andrews LB, et al: An alternative strategy for studying adverse events in medical care. *Lancet* 349(9048):309–13, 1997.

Armstrong EP, Chrischilles EA: Electronic prescribing and monitoring are needed to improve drug usc. *Arch Int Med* 160:2713–4, 9 Oct 2000.

Bates DW: A 40-year-old woman who noticed a medication error. *JAMA* 285:3134–40, 27 Jun 2001.

Bates DW, et al: The impact of computerized physician order entry on medication error prevention. *J Am Med Inform Assoc* 6(4):313–21, 1999.

Bates DW, et al: Effect of computerized physician order entry and a team intervention on prevention of serious medication errors. *JAMA* 280(15):1311–6, 1998.

Bates DW, et al: Incidence of adverse drug events and potential adverse drug events. *JAMA* 274(1):29–34, 1995.

Battles JB, Shea CE: A system of analyzing medical errors to improve GME curricula and programs. *Academic Medicine* 76:125–33, Feb 2001.

Berry MC: The good things about telling the truth: A discussion about disclosing health care errors. Presented at the Annenberg IV conference, Indianapolis, IN, 23 Apr 2002.

Berwick DM, et al: Reducing adverse drug events and medical errors. Presented at the National Forum on Quality Improvement in Health Care Conference, New Orleans, LA, 4–7 Dec 1996.

Beyers M (ed): *The Business of Nursing.* Chicago: American Hospital Publishing, 1996.

Binius T: Ability to prescribe on-line growing faster than acceptance. *Am Medical News* 20 April 1998.

Blumenthal D: Making medical errors into medical treasures. *JAMA* 272(23):1851–7, 1994.

Bogner MS (ed): *Human Error in Medicine.* Hillsdale, NJ: Lawrence Erlbaum Associates, 1994.

Bradshaw BG, Liu SS, Thirlby RC: Standardized perioperative care protocols and reduced length of stay after colon surgery. *J Am Coll Surg* 186(5):501–6, 1998.

Brennan TA: The Institute of Medicine Report on medical errors—Could it do harm? *NEJM* 342:1123–5, 13 Apr 2000.

Brennan TA, et al: Incidence of adverse events and negligence in hospitalized patients: Results of the Harvard Medical Practice Study I. *NEJM* 324:370–6, 7 Feb 1991.

Busch KA, et al: Clinical features of inpatient suicide. *Psych Annals* 23(5):256–62, 1993.

Byington M, Bender A: Commentary: Communicating with patients. *Forum* 20:1–2, Dec 2000.

Cardell R, Horton-Deutsch SL: A model for assessment of inpatient suicide potential. *Arch Psychiatr Nurs* 8(6):366–72, 1994.

Cardell R, Quinnett P, Bratcher K: *QPRT-II Suicide Risk Management Inventory—Hospital Version.* Spokane, WA: Cardell, Quinnett, and Bratcher, 1999.

Carthey J, et al: Human factors and cardiac surgery: Identifying problems and positive aspects of surgical performance. Presented at Enhancing Patient Safety and Reducing Errors in Health Care (Annenberg II), Rancho Mirage, CA, 9 Nov 1998.

Chassin MR, Becher EC: The wrong patient. *Ann Intern Med* 136:826–33, Jun 2002.

Clark PA: What residents are not learning: Observations in an NICU. *Acad Med* 76:419–24, May 2001.

Cohen MR (ed): *Medication Errors.* Washington, DC: American Pharmaceutical Association, 1999.

Cole T: Medical errors vs medical injuries: Physicians seek to prevent both. *JAMA* 284:2175–7, 1 Nov 2000.

Cook RI: Two years before the mast: Learning how to learn about patient safety. Presented at Enhancing Patient Safety and Reducing Errors in Health Care (Annenberg II), Rancho Mirage, CA, 8–10 Nov 1998.

Cook RI, Woods DD: Operating at the sharp end: The complexity of human error. In Bogner MS (ed): *Human Error in Medicine.* Hillsdale, NJ: Lawrence Erlbaum Associates, 1994.

Cooper JB, et al: Effects of information feedback and pulse oximetry on the incidence of anesthesia complications. *Anesthesiology* 67(5):686–94, 1987.

Coulter A: Partnerships with patients: The pros and cons of shared clinical decision-making. *J Health Serv Res Policy* 2:112–21, Apr 1997.

Darr K: Uncircling the wagons: Informing patients about unanticipated outcomes. *Hosp Topics* 79:33–5, Summer 2001.

Dwyer K: Multiple systems breakdowns. *Forum* 21:19, Summer 2001.

Dwyer K: Surgery-related claims and the systems involved. *Forum* 21:1–4, Summer 2001.

Engaging physicians in the performance improvement process. *Jt Comm Persp* 21:8–9, Jul 2001.

Evans LK, Strumpf NE: Myths about elder restraint. *J Nurs Scholarship* 22:124–8, Summer 1990.

Evans LK, Strumpf NE: Tying down the elderly. *J Am Geriatr Soc* 37(1):65–74, 1989.

Evans LK, Strumpf NE, Williams C: Redefining a standard of care for frail older people: Alternatives to routine physical restraint. In Katz P, Kane R, Mezey R (eds): *Advances in Long Term Care*. New York: Springer, 1991.

Evans RS, et al: A computer-assisted management program for antibiotics and other antiinfective agents. *NEJM* 338:232–8, 22 Jan 1998.

Farberow NL: Guidelines to suicide prevention in the hospital. In Shneidman ES, Farberow NL, Litman RL (eds): *The Psychology of Suicide: A Clinician's Guide to Evaluation and Treatment.* Northvale, NJ: J. Aronson, 1994.

Fisher WA: Restraint and seclusion: A review of the literature. *Am J Psychiatry* 151:1584–91, Nov 1994.

Fletcher K: Use of restraints in the elderly. *AACN Clinical Issues* 7:611–20, Nov 1996.

Forrest J, et al: Multicenter study of general anesthesia. II. Results. *Anesthesiology* 72(2):262–8, 1990.

Frank C, Hodgetts G, Puxty J: Safety and efficacy of physical restraints for the elderly. *Can Fam Physician* 42:2402–9, Dec 1996.

Gaba DM: Anaesthesiology as a model for patient safety in health care. *BMJ* 320:785–8, 18 Mar 2000.

Gandhi TK, et al: Drug complications in outpatients. *J Gen Intern Med* 15:149–54, Mar 2000.

Gosbee J, Stahlhut R: Teaching medical students and residents about error in health care. Presented at Enhancing Patient Safety and Reducing Errors in Health Care (Annenberg I), Rancho Mirage, CA, Oct 1996.

Greengold NL: A Web-based program for implementing evidence-based patient safety recommendations. *Jt Comm J Qual Improv* 28:340–8, Jun 2002.

Hanlon JT, et al: A randomized, controlled trial of a clinical pharmacist intervention to improve inappropriate prescribing in elderly outpatients with polypharmacy. *Am J Med* 100(4):428–37, 1996.

Harbison S, Regehr G: Faculty and resident opinions regarding the role of morbidity and mortality conference. *Am J Surg* 177:136–9, Feb 1999.

Haugh R: To the rescue. *Hosp Health Network,* pp 44–8, Apr 2000.

Hebert PC: Disclosure of adverse events and errors in healthcare: An ethical perspective. *Drug Safety* 24(15):1095–1104.

Hepler CD, Strand LM: Opportunities and responsibilities in pharmaceutical care. *Am J Hosp Pharm* 47:533–43, Mar 1990.

Hingorani M, Wong T, Vafidis G: Patients' and doctors' attitudes to amount of information given after unintended injury during treatment: Cross sectional, questionnaire survey. *BMJ* 318:640–1, 6 Mar 1999.

Hofer TP, Kerr EA, Hayward RA: What is an error? *Eff Clin Pract* 3:261–9, Nov/Dec 2000.

Hyman WA: Errors in the use of medical equipment. In Bogner MS (ed): *Human Error in Medicine.* Hillsdale, NJ: Lawrence Erlbaum Associates, 1994.

Institute of Medicine: *Crossing the Quality Chasm: A New Health System for the 21st Century.* Washington, DC: National Academy Press, 2001.

Institute of Medicine: *To Err Is Human: Building a Safer Health System.* Washington, DC: National Academy Press, 2000.

Jacobs DG (ed): *The Harvard Medical School Guide to Suicide Assessment and Intervention.* San Francisco: Jossey-Bass, 1999.

Johns MME: The time has come to reform graduate medical education. *JAMA* 286:1075–6, 5 Sep 2001.

Jones FG, Hallman C: Creating a culture of safety. Presented at CSR Orion II, Atlanta, Jan 2002.

Kaiser Family Foundation and the Agency for Healthcare Research and Quality: *National Survey on Americans as Health Care Consumers: An Update on the Role of Quality Information.* Menlo Park, CA, Dec 2000. Web site: www.kff.org.

Ketring SP, White JP: Developing a systemwide approach to patient safety. *Jt Comm J Qual Improv* 28:287–95, Jun 2002.

Knox GE, et al: Downsizing, reengineering and patient safety: Numbers, new-ness and resultant risk. *J Health Risk Manag* 19:18–25, Fall 1999.

Kraman SS, Hamm G: Risk management: Extreme honesty may be the best policy. *Ann Intern Med* 131:963–7, 21 Dec 1999.

Krizek TJ: Surgical error: Ethical issues of adverse events. *Arch Surg* 135:1359–66, Nov 2000.

Kuperman GJ, et al: Patient safety and computerized medication ordering at Brigham and Women's Hospital. *J Qual Improve* 27:509–21, Oct 2001.

Lamberg L: Long hours, little sleep: Bad medicine for physicians-in-training? *JAMA* 287:303–6, 16 Jan 2002.

Leape LL, Berwick DM, Bates DW: What practices will most improve safety? Evidence-based medicine meets patient safety. *JAMA* 288:501–7, 24/31 Jul 2002.

Leape LL, et al: Pharmacist participation on physician rounds and adverse drug events in the intensive care unit. *JAMA* 282(3):267–70, 1999.

Leape LL, et al: Promoting patient safety by preventing medical error. *JAMA* 280, 28 Oct 1998.

Leape LL, et al: The nature of adverse events in hospitalized patients: Results of the Harvard Medical Practice Study II. *NEJM* 324:377–84, 7 Feb 1991.

Lesar TS, Briceland L, Stein DS: Factors related to errors in medication prescribing. *JAMA* 277(4):312–7, 1997.

Lester H, Tritter JQ: Medical error: A discussion of the medical construction of error and suggestions for reforms of medical education to decrease error. *Medical Education* 35:855–61, Sep 2001.

Levine JM: Historical notes on restraint reduction: The legacy of Dr. Philippe Pinel. *J Am Ger Soc* 44:1130–3, Sep 1996.

Lin B, Anderson LR: The role of the pharmacy department in the prevention of adverse drug events: A survey of current practices. *Pharm Pract Manage Q* 17(1):10–6, 1997.

Litman RE: Suicide prevention in a treatment setting. *Suicide Life Threat Behav* 25(1):134–42, 1995.

Martin PB: Using closed malpractice claims as teaching tools. *Forum* 18:1, Mar 1998.

Mathias JM: VHA's program to curb wrong-site surgery. *OR Manager* 18:7–9, Mar 2002.

Mawji Z, et al: First do no harm: Integrating patient safety and quality improvement. *Jt Comm J Qual Improv* 28:373–86, Jul 2002.

Medication safety issue brief 5: Crucial role of therapeutic guidelines. *Hosp Health Netw* 75:65–6, May 2001.

Mello MM: Commentary: The role of clinical practice guidelines in malpractice litigation. *Forum* 20:1, Fall 2000.

Meltzer B: Wrong site surgery: Are your patients at risk? *Outpatient Surgery Magazine* 111:26–35, Feb 2002.

Merr A, Smith AM: *Errors, Medicine, and the Law.* Cambridge, UK: Cambridge University Press, 2001.

Meyer TA: Improving the quality of the order-writing process for inpatient orders and outpatient prescriptions. *Am J Health-Syst Pharm* 57 (Suppl 4): S18–S22, 15 Dec 2000.

Midwest Medical Insurance Company: Risk Management Advisory. Minneapolis, 1997.

Miller CF, Dolter KJ: Evidence-based condition management: DoD/VA clinical practice guidelines—Tools to effect best practices. Presented at the 2001 TRICARE conference, Washington, DC, 24 Jan 2001.

Montazeri M, Cook DJ: Impact of a clinical pharmacist in a multidisciplinary intensive care unit. *Crit Care Med* 22:1044 8, Jun 1994.

Moray N: Error reduction as a systems problem. In Bogner MS (ed): *Human Error in Medicine.* Hillsdale, NJ: Lawrence Erlbaum Associates, 1994.

Murayama KM, et al: A critical evaluation of the morbidity and mortality conference. *Am J Surg* 183:246–50, Mar 2002.

Nadzam DM: A systems approach to medication use. In Cousins DD (ed): *Medication Use: A Systems Approach to Reducing Errors.* Oakbrook Terrace, IL: Joint Commission, 1998.

National Coordinating Council for Medication Error Reporting and Prevention: About medication errors. Web site: www.nccmerp.org/aboutmederrors.htm.

National Patient Safety Foundation at the American Medical Association: *Public Opinion of Patient Safety Issues: Research Findings.* Sep 1997. Web site: www.npsf.org.

Newcomer LN: Medicare pharmacy coverage: Ensuring safety before funding. *Health Affairs* 19:59–62, Mar/Apr 2000.

O'Leary DS: Statement of the Joint Commission on Accreditation of Healthcare Organizations before the House Committee on Energy and Commerce Subcommittee on Health, 8 May 2002.

O'Leary DS: Editorial: Accreditation's role in reducing medical errors. *British Medical Journal* 320:727–28, Mar 2000.

O'Leary DS: Statement of the Joint Commission on Accreditation of Healthcare Organizations before the Committee on Health, Education, Labor and Pensions, U.S. Senate and the Subcommittee on Labor, Health and Human Services, and Education of the Senate Committee on Appropriations, 22 Feb 2000.

Owens MF: Patient restraints: Protection for whom? *JONA's Healthcare Law, Ethics, and Reg* 2:59–65, Jun 2000.

Porto GG: Disclosure of medical error: Facts and fallacies. *J Healthcare Risk Manage* 21:71–6, Fall 2001.

Proulx S, Wilfinger R, Cohen MR: Medication error prevention: Profiling one of pharmacy's foremost advocacy efforts for advice on error prevention. *Pharm Pract Manage Q* 17(1):1–9, 1997.

Puopolo AL, Brennan TA: The value of improving test result communication. *Forum* 20:13–4, Feb 2000.

Quality Interagency Coordination Task Force: *Doing what counts for patient safety: Federal actions to reduce medical errors and their impact.* Report to the President, Feb 2000. Web site: www.quic.gov

Raish DW: Patient counseling in community pharmacy and its relationship with prescription payment methods and practice settings. *Ann Pharmacother* 27(10):1173–9, 1993.

Reason J: *Human Error.* Cambridge, UK: Cambridge University Press, 1990.

Risk Management Foundation: A conversation with Lucian Leape, MD. *Forum* 21:5–7, Summer 2001.

Rosenthal MM, Sutcliffe KM (eds): *Medical Error: What Do We Know? What Do We Do?* San Francisco: Jossey-Bass, 2002.

Rosner F, et al: Disclosure and prevention of medical errors. *Arch Intern Med* 160(14):2089–92, 24 Jul 2000.

Sarrouf C: Narrow diagnostic focus: A plaintiff attorney's perspective. *Forum* 18:15, May 2002.

Scherer YK, et al: The nursing dilemma of restraints. *J Ger Nurs* 17:14–7, Feb 1991.

Schiff GD, Rucker TD: Computerized prescribing: Building the electronic infrastructure for better medication usage. *JAMA* 279(13):1024–9, 1998.

Sharpe VA: "No tribunal other than his own conscience": Historical reflections on harm and responsibility in medicine. Presented at Enhancing Patient Safety and Reducing Errors in Health Care (Annenberg II), Rancho Mirage, CA, 8 Nov 1998.

Shelton JD: The harm of "First, do no harm." *JAMA* 284:2687–8, 6 Dec 2000.

Shojania K, et al (eds): *Making Health Care Safer: A Critical Analysis of Patient Safety Practices.* Rockville, MD: Agency for Healthcare Research and Quality Web site: www.ahrq.gov/clinic/ptsafety.

Shojania KG, et al: Safe but sound: Patient safety meets evidence-based medicine. *JAMA* 288:508–13, 24/31 Jul 2002.

Small SD: Principles for developing education and training to improve patient safety. *Forum* 21:10–2, Summer 2001.

Smetzer J: Prescriptions for safety. *AHA News* 20 Mar 2000.

Spath PL (ed): *Error Reduction in Health Care: A Systems Approach to Improving Patient Safety.* San Francisco: Jossey-Bass, 2000.

Spencer FC: Human error in hospitals and industrial accidents: Current concepts. *J Am Coll Surg* 191:410–8, Oct 2000.

Strumpf NE, Evans LK: Alternatives to physical restraints. *J Ger Nurs* 18(11):4, 1992.

Strumpf NE, Evans LK: The ethical problems of prolonged physical restraint. *J Ger Nurs* 17:27–30, Feb 1991.

Studdert DM, Brennan TA: No-fault compensation for medical injuries: The prospect for error prevention. *JAMA* 286:217–23, 11 Jul 2001.

Sullivan-Marx EM: Physical and chemical restraints: Meeting the challenge. *Dimensions of Crit Care Nurs* 13:58–9, Mar/Apr 1994.

Thornton PD, Simon S, Mathew TH: Towards safer drug prescribing, dispensing and administration in hospitals. *J Qual Clin Practice* 19:41–5, Mar 1999.

Tinetti M, Liu W, Ginter S: Mechanical restraint use and fall-related injuries among residents of skilled nursing facilities. *Ann Intern Med* 116(5):369–74, 1992.

Tinker JH, et al: Role of monitoring devices in prevention of anesthetic mishaps: A closed claims analysis. *Anesthesiology* 71:541–6, Oct 1989.

U.S. Food and Drug Administration: Improving public health: Promoting safe and effective drug use. Web site: www.fda.gov/opacom/factsheets/justthefacts/3cder.html.

Usherwood T: Subjective and behavioural evaluation of the teaching of patient interview skills. *Med Educ* 27:41–7, Jan 1993.

VanCott H: Human errors: Their causes and reduction. In Bogner MS (ed): *Human Error in Medicine.* Hillsdale, NJ: Lawrence Erlbaum Associates, 1994.

Vincent CA, et al: Why do people sue doctors? A study of patients and relatives taking legal action. *Lancet* 343:1609–13, 25 Jun 1994.

Voelker R: Hospital collaborative creates tools to help reduce medication errors. *JAMA* 286:3067–9, 26 Dec 2001.

Weingart SN, et al: A physician-based voluntary reporting system for adverse events and medical errors. *J Gen Int Med* 16:809–14, Dec 2001.

Werner P, et al: Individualized care alternatives used in the process of removing physical restraints in the nursing home. *J Am Geriatr Soc* 42:321–5, Mar 1994.

White MK: Patient adherence. Presented at the Medication Errors Symposium, Baltimore, MD, 7–8 Apr 2000.

Witman AB, Park DM, Hardin SB: How do patients want physicians to handle mistakes? A survey of internal medicine patients in an academic setting. *Arch Intern Med* 156:2565–9, 9–23 Dec 1996.

Wu AW: Medical error: The second victim: The doctor who makes the mistake needs help too. *BMJ* 320:726–7, 18 Mar 2000.

Wu AW: Handling hospital errors: Is disclosure the best defense? *Ann Intern Med* 131:970–2, 21 Dec 1999.

Wu AW, et al: To tell the truth: Ethical and practical issues in disclosing medical mistakes to patients. *J Gen Int Med* 12:770–5, Dec 1997.

Wu AW, et al: Do house officers learn from their mistakes? *JAMA* 265(16):2089–94, 1991.

Xiao Y, Seagull J: Toward a user friendly health care environment: The case of alarms. *Forum* 21:17–8, Summer 2001.

Safety and Health Care Error Reduction Standards*

Patient Rights and Organization Ethics (RI)

Standard RI.1.2.2
Patients and, when appropriate, their families are informed about the outcomes of care, including unanticipated outcomes.

Intent of RI.1.2.2
At a minimum, the patient and, when appropriate, the patient's family are informed about

- outcomes of care that the patient (or family) must be knowledgeable about in order to participate in current and future decisions affecting the patient's care; and
- unanticipated outcomes of care that relate to sentinel events considered reviewable by the Joint Commission. The responsible licensed independent practitioner (LIP) or his or her designee informs the patient (and when appropriate, the patient's family) about these outcomes of care.

Education (PF)

Standard PF.3.7
Education includes information about patient responsibilities in the patient's care.

Intent of PF.3.7
The safety of health care delivery is enhanced by the involvement of the patient, as appropriate to his/her condition, as a partner in the health care process. In addition, hospitals are entitled to reasonable and responsible behavior on the part of the patients and their families. The hospital identifies patient and family responsibilities and educates the patient and

family about these responsibilities. Specific attention is directed at educating patients and families about their role in helping to facilitate the safe delivery of care.

Responsibilities include at least the following:
- Providing information. The patient is responsible for providing, to the best of his or her knowledge, accurate and complete information about present complaints, past illnesses, hospitalizations, medications, and other matters relating to his or her health. The patient and family are responsible for reporting perceived risks in their care and unexpected changes in the patient's condition. The patient and family help the hospital improve its understanding of the patient's environment by providing feedback about service needs and expectations.
- Asking questions. Patients are responsible for asking questions when they do not understand what they have been told about their care or what they are expected to do.
- Following instructions. The patient and family are responsible for following the care, service, or treatment plan developed. They should express any concerns they have about their ability to follow and comply with the proposed care plan or course of treatment. Every effort is made to adapt the plan to the patient's specific needs and limitations. When such adaptations to the treatment plan are not recommended, the patient and family are responsible for

---

* This version of the safety and health care error reduction standards appears in the *Comprehensive Accreditation Manual for Hospitals (CAMH)*. Similar standards appear in manuals of other programs.

understanding the consequences of the treatment alternatives and not following the proposed course.

- Accepting consequences. The patient and family are responsible for the outcomes if they do not follow the care, service, or treatment plan.
- Following rules and regulations. The patient and family are responsible for following the hospital's rules and regulations concerning patient care and conduct.
- Showing respect and consideration. Patients and families are responsible for being considerate of the hospital's personnel and property.
- Meeting financial commitments. The patient and family are responsible for promptly meeting any financial obligation agreed to with the hospital.

Patients are educated about their responsibilities during the admission, registration, or intake process and as needed thereafter.

The patient's family or surrogate decision-maker assumes the above responsibility for the patient if the patient has been found by his or her physician to be incapable of understanding these responsibilities, has been judged incompetent in accordance with law, or exhibits a communication barrier.

The hospital informs each patient of his or her responsibilities either verbally, in writing, or both, based on hospital policy.

Patients are responsible for being considerate of other patients, helping control noise and disturbances, following smoking policies, and respecting others' property.

Continuum of Care (CC)

Standard CC.3.1
The hospital provides for coordination of care and services among health professionals and settings.

Intent of CC.3.1
Communication and transfer of information between and among the care professionals and settings is essential to a seamless, safe, and effective process.

The patient frequently may require more than one service from a hospital. The hospital ensures that such care or services are coordinated among staff, whether provided directly or through written agreement. This minimizes the potential for missed, conflicting, or duplicated services. If the hospital is aware of duplication or conflict, it attempts to correct the situation.

Improving Organization Performance (PI)

Standard PI.2
New or modified processes are designed well.

Intent of PI.2
When processes, functions, or services are designed well, they draw on a variety of information sources. Good process design

a. is consistent with the organization's mission, vision, values, goals and objectives, and plans;
b. meets the needs of individuals served, staff, and others;
c. is clinically sound and current (for instance, use of practice guidelines, successful practices, information from relevant literature, and clinical standards);
d. is consistent with sound business practices;
e. incorporates available information from within the organization and from other organizations about potential risks to patients, including the occurrence of sentinel events in order to minimize risks to patients affected by the new or redesigned process, function, or service;
f. includes analysis and/or pilot testing to determine whether the proposed design/redesign is an improvement; and
g. incorporates the results of performance improvement activities.

The organization incorporates information related to these elements, when available and relevant, in the design or redesign of processes, functions, or services.

Standard PI.3

Data are collected to monitor the stability of existing processes, identify opportunities for improvement, identify changes that will lead to improvement, and sustain improvement.

Intent of PI.3

Collected data help the organization evaluate outcomes or determine the performance of a function or process. When data collection is systematic, it can be used to

- establish a performance baseline;
- describe process performance or stability;
- describe the dimensions of performance relevant to functions, processes, and outcomes;
- identify areas for more focused data collection; and
- sustain improvement.

The leaders use the judgments made about stability or performance to identify and prioritize issues for more focused data collection and analysis (see LD.1.4, LD.4.2, and LD.4.3 for the leaders using criteria to prioritize data collection for improvement).

Standard PI.4.3

Undesirable patterns or trends in performance and sentinel events are intensively analyzed.

Intent of PI.4.3

When the organization detects or suspects significant undesirable performance or variation, it initiates intense analysis to determine where best to focus changes for improvement. The organization initiates intense analysis when the comparisons show that

- levels of performance, patterns, or trends vary significantly and undesirably from those expected;
- performance varies significantly and undesirably from that of other organizations;

- performance varies significantly and undesirably from recognized standards; or
- a sentinel event has occurred.

When monitoring performance of specific clinical processes, certain events always elicit intense analysis. Based on the scope of care or services provided, intense analysis is performed for the following:

- Confirmed transfusion reactions;
- Significant adverse drug reactions;
- Significant medication errors;
- Hazardous conditions; and
- Staffing effectiveness issues.

Intense analysis should also occur for those topics chosen by the leaders as performance improvement priorities and priorities for proactive reduction in patient risk (see LD.1.4 and LD.5.2), or when undesirable variation occurs that changes the priorities. Intense analysis involves studying a process to learn in greater detail about how it is performed or how it operates, how it can malfunction, and how errors occur.

A root cause analysis is performed when a sentinel event occurs. An intense analysis is also performed for the following:

- Major discrepancies, or patterns of discrepancies, between preoperative and postoperative (including pathologic) diagnoses, including those identified during the pathologic review of specimens removed during surgical or invasive procedures; and
- Significant adverse events associated with anesthesia use.

Standard PI.4.4

The organization identifies changes that will lead to improved performance and improve patient safety.

Intent of PI.4.4

The organization uses the information from the data analysis to identify system changes that will improve performance or improve patient safety.

Changes are identified based on the analysis of data from targeted study or from analysis of data from ongoing monitoring. A change is selected, and the organization plans to implement the change on a pilot test basis or across the organization. Performance measures are selected that help determine the effectiveness of the change and whether it resulted in an improvement (see PI.3.1.1, PI.3.1.2, and PI.3.1.3) once the change is implemented.

Leadership (LD)

Standard LD.1.4

The planning process provides for setting performance improvement priorities and identifies how the hospital adjusts priorities in response to unusual or urgent events.

Intent of LD.1.4

The planning process provides the framework or criteria for establishing performance improvement priorities. The planning process gives priority consideration to:

- Processes that affect a large percentage of patients;
- Processes that place patients at risk if not performed well, if performed when not indicated, or if not performed when indicated; and
- Processes that have been or are likely to be problem prone.

The hospital's priority setting is sensitive to emerging needs such as those identified through data collection and assessment, unanticipated adverse occurrences affecting patients, changing regulatory requirements, significant patient and staff needs, changes in the environment of care, or changes in the community.

Standard LD.1.8

The leaders and other relevant personnel collaborate in decision making.

Intent of LD.1.8

The hospital's leaders and directors of relevant departments collaborate in

- development of hospitalwide patient care programs, policies, and procedures that describe how patients' care needs are assessed and met;
- development and implementation of the hospital's plan for providing patient care;
- decision-making structures and processes; and
- implementation of an effective and continuous program to measure, assess, and improve performance and improve safety.

Standard LD.3.2

The leaders foster communication and coordination among individuals and departments.

Intent of LD.3.2

To coordinate and integrate patient care and improve patient safety, the leaders develop a culture that emphasizes cooperation and communication. An open communication system facilitates an interdisciplinary approach to providing patient care. The leaders develop methods for promoting communication among services, individual staff members, and less formal structures such as quality action teams, performance improvement teams, or members of standing committees.

This leadership role is commonly referred to as coaching.

Standard LD.3.4.1

The leaders provide for mechanisms to measure, analyze, and manage variation in the performance of defined processes that affect patient safety.

Intent of LD.3.4.1

Inconsistency in the performance of processes, as intended by their design and described in organization policies and procedures, frequently leads to unanticipated and undesirable results. In order to minimize risk to patients due to such variation, the leaders ensure that the actual performance of processes identified as error prone or high risk regarding patient safety is measured and analyzed, and when significant variation is identified, appropriate corrective actions are taken to enhance the system(s).

At any given time, the performance of critical steps in at least one high-risk process is the subject of ongoing measurement and periodic analysis to determine the degree of variation from intended performance.

Standard LD.4.4

The leaders allocate adequate resources for measuring, assessing, and improving the hospital's performance and for improving patient safety.

Standard LD.4.4.1

The leaders assign personnel needed to participate in performance improvement activities and activities to improve patient safety.

Standard LD.4.4.2

The leaders provide adequate time for personnel to participate in performance improvement activities and activities to improve patient safety.

Standard LD.4.4.3

The leaders provide information systems and data management processes for ongoing performance improvement and improvement of patient safety.

Standard LD.4.4.4

The leaders provide for staff training in the basic approaches to and methods of performance improvement and improvement of patient safety.

Standard LD.4.4.5

The leaders assess the adequacy of their allocation of human, information, physical, and financial resources in support of their identified performance improvement and safety improvement priorities.

Intent of LD.4.4 Through LD.4.4.5

Hospital leaders provide adequate human resources for these activities and give them sufficient time and

support to be effective. Appropriate staff members are assigned in sufficient numbers to ensure progress in the pursuit of improvement priorities and risk-reduction priorities. Leaders allow enough time for performance improvement activities and activities to improve patient safety and provide needed information and technical assistance. Each department determines what resources are sufficient for its improvement efforts and activities to improve patient safety.

Standard LD.4.5

The leaders measure and assess the effectiveness of their contributions to improving performance and improving patient safety.

Intent of LD.4.5

The performance improvement framework in the "Improving Organization Performance" chapter is used to design, measure, assess, and improve the leaders' performance and contribution to performance improvement and improvement in patient safety.

The leaders

- set measurable objectives for improving hospital performance and improving patient safety;
- gather information to assess their effectiveness in improving hospital performance and in improving patient safety;
- use pre-established, objective process criteria to assess their effectiveness in improving hospital performance and in improving patient safety;
- draw conclusions based on their findings and develop and implement improvement in their activities; and
- evaluate their performance to support sustained improvement.

INTRODUCTION TO PATIENT SAFETY AND MEDICAL/HEALTH CARE ERRORS REDUCTION STANDARDS

Standards throughout this manual are designed to improve patient safety and reduce risk to patients.

Recognizing that effective medical/health care error reduction requires an integrated and coordinated approach, the following standards relate specifically to leadership's role in an organizationwide safety program that includes all activities within the organization which contribute to the maintenance and improvement of patient safety, such as performance improvement, environmental safety, and risk management. The standards do not require the creation of new structures or "offices" within the organization; rather, the standards emphasize the need to integrate all patient-safety activities, both existing and newly created, with an identified locus of accountability within the organization's leadership.

Although the standards focus on patient safety, it would be difficult to create an organizationwide safety initiative that excludes staff and visitors. Furthermore, many of the activities taken to improve patient safety (such as, security, equipment safety, infection control) encompass staff and visitors as well as patients.

Effective reduction of medical/health care errors and other factors that contribute to unintended adverse patient outcomes in a health care organization requires an environment in which patients, their families, and organization staff and leaders can identify and manage actual and potential risks to patient safety. This environment encourages recognition and acknowledgment of risks to patient safety and medical/health care errors; the initiation of actions to reduce these risks; the internal reporting of what has been found and the actions taken; a focus on processes and systems; and minimization of individual blame or retribution for involvement in a medical/health care error. It encourages organizational learning about medical/health care errors and supports the sharing of that knowledge to effect behavioral changes in itself and other health care organizations to improve patient safety. The leaders of the organization are responsible for fostering such an environment through their personal example and by establishing

mechanisms that support effective responses to actual occurrences; ongoing proactive reduction in medical/health care errors; and integration of patient safety priorities into the new design and redesign of all relevant organization processes, functions, and services.

Standard LD.5

The leaders ensure implementation of an integrated patient safety program throughout the organization.

Intent of LD.5

The patient safety program includes at least the following:

- Designation of one or more qualified individuals or an interdisciplinary group to manage the organizationwide patient safety program. Typically these individuals may include directors of performance improvement, safety officers, risk managers, and clinical leaders.
- Definition of the scope of the program activities, that is, the types of occurrences to be addressed—typically ranging from "no harm" frequently occurring "slips" to sentinel events with serious adverse outcomes.
- Description of mechanisms to ensure that all components of the health care organization are integrated into and participate in the organizationwide program.
- Procedures for immediate response to medical/health care errors, including care of the affected patient(s), containment of risk to others, and preservation of factual information for subsequent analysis.
- Clear systems for internal and external reporting of information relating to medical/health care errors.
- Defined mechanisms for responding to the various types of occurrences, such as, root cause analysis in response to a sentinel event, or for conducting proactive risk reduction activities.
- Defined mechanisms for support of staff who have been involved in a sentinel event.
- At least annually, a report to the governing

body on the occurrence of medical/health care errors and actions taken to improve patient safety, both in response to actual occurrences and proactively.

Standard LD.5.1

Leaders ensure that the processes for identifying and managing sentinel events are defined and implemented.

Intent of LD.5.1

When a sentinel event occurs in a health care organization, it is necessary that appropriate individuals within the organization be aware of the event; investigate and understand the causes that underlie the event; and make changes in the organization's systems and processes to reduce the probability of such an event in the future. The leaders are responsible for establishing processes for the identification, reporting, analysis, and prevention of sentinel events and for ensuring the consistent and effective implementation of a mechanism to accomplish these activities including

- determination of a definition of sentinel event, which is approved by the leaders and communicated throughout the organization. At a minimum, the organization's definition of sentinel event must include those events that are subject to review under the Joint Commission's Sentinel Event Policy as published in this manual and may include near misses;
- creation of a process for reporting of sentinel events through established channels within the organization and, as appropriate, to external agencies in accordance with law and regulation;
- creation of a process for conducting thorough and credible root cause analyses that focuses on process and system factors; and
- documentation of a risk-reduction strategy and action plan that includes measurement of the effectiveness of process and system improvements to reduce risk.

Standard LD.5.2

Leaders ensure that an ongoing, proactive program for identifying risks to patient safety and reducing medical/health care errors is defined and implemented.

Intent of LD.5.2

The organization seeks to reduce the risk of sentinel events and medical/health care system error-related occurrences by conducting its own proactive risk assessment activities and by using available information about sentinel events known to occur in health care organizations that provide similar care and services. This effort is undertaken so that processes, functions, and services can be designed or redesigned to prevent such occurrences in the organization. Proactive identification and management of potential risks to patient safety have the obvious advantage of preventing adverse occurrences, rather than simply reacting when they occur. This approach also avoids the barriers to understanding created by hindsight bias and the fear of disclosure, embarrassment, blame, and punishment that can arise in the wake of an actual event.

Leaders provide direction and resources to conduct the following proactive activities to reduce risk to patients:

- At least annually, select at least one high-risk process for proactive risk assessment; such selection is to be based, in part, on information published periodically by the Joint Commission that identifies the most frequently occurring types of sentinel events and patient safety risk factors;
- Assess the intended and actual implementation of the process to identify the steps in the process where there is, or may be, undesirable variation (what engineers call potential "failure modes");
- For each identified "failure mode" identify the possible effects on patients (what engineers call the "effect"), and how serious the possible effect on the patient could be (what engineers call the "criticality" of the effect);

- For the most critical effects, conduct a root cause analysis to determine why the variation (the failure mode) leading to that effect may occur;
- Redesign the process and/or underlying systems to minimize the risk of that failure mode or to protect patients from the effects of that failure mode;
- Test and implement the redesigned process;
- Identify and implement measures of the effectiveness of the redesigned process; and
- Implement a strategy for maintaining the effectiveness of the redesigned process over time.

Standard LD.5.3

Leaders ensure that patient safety issues are given a high priority and addressed when processes, functions, or services are designed or redesigned.

Intent of LD.5.3

When processes, functions, or services are designed or redesigned, information from within the organization and from other organizations about potential risks to patient safety, including the occurrence of sentinel events, is considered and, where appropriate, used to minimize the risk to patients affected by the new or redesigned process, function, or service.

Management of Human Resources (HR)

Standard HR.4

An orientation process provides initial job training and information and assesses the staff's ability to fulfill specified responsibilities.

Intent of HR.4

The orientation process assesses each staff member's ability to fulfill specific responsibilities. The process familiarizes staff members with their jobs and with the work environment before the staff begins patient care or other activities. In this way, the process promotes safe and effective job performance. The orientation process emphasizes specific job-related aspects of patient safety. When the hospital uses

volunteer services, volunteers are oriented to patient care, safety, infection control, and any other activities they are expected to perform competently.

Standard HR.4.2

Ongoing in-service and other education and training maintain and improve staff competence and support an interdisciplinary approach to patient care.

Intent of HR.4.2

The hospital ensures that each staff member participates in ongoing in-service education and other training to increase his or her knowledge of work-related issues. Ongoing in-service and other education and training programs emphasize specific job-related aspects of patient safety. As appropriate, this training incorporates methods of team training to foster an interdisciplinary, collaborative approach to the delivery of patient care, and reinforces the need and way(s) to report medical/health care errors. The hospital periodically reviews the staff's abilities to carry out job responsibilities, especially when introducing new procedures, techniques, technology, and equipment. Ongoing in-service and other education and training programs are appropriate to patient age groups served by the hospital.

Management of Information (IM)

Standard IM.1

The hospital plans and designs information management processes to meet internal and external information needs.

Intent of IM.1

Hospitals vary in size, complexity, governance, structure, decision-making processes, and resources. Information management systems and processes vary accordingly. An information system consists of effective methodologies to maintain and process data. Although computer-based information is often referenced when considering information processing and management, it is understood that data also consist of written, pictorial, graphic, and spoken forms, for which information management systems are used to manage and continuously improve care and organizational processes.

The hospital bases its information management processes on a thorough analysis of internal and external information needs. The analysis ascertains the flow of information in a hospital, including information storage and feedback mechanisms. The analysis considers what data and information are needed within and among departments, services, or programs, the clinical staff, the administration, and governance structure, as well as information needed to support relationships with outside services, contractors, companies, and agencies. The hospital bases management, staffing, and material resource allocations for information management on the scope and complexity of services provided. Leaders seek input from staff in information needs, selecting appropriate information technology, and integrating and using information systems to manage clinical and organizational information. Appropriate staff and leaders ensure that required data and information are provided efficiently for individual care, research, education, and management at every level.

The hospital assesses its information management needs based on its
- mission;
- goals;
- services;
- personnel;
- mode(s) of service delivery;
- resources;
- access to affordable technology; and
- identification of barriers to effective communication among caregivers.

The hospital also considers its information needs for
- licensing, accrediting, and regulatory bodies;
- purchasers, payers, and employers; and
- participation in national research and care databases.

This analysis guides development of processes for managing information used internally and externally.

When the hospital assesses its overall information needs, it also looks at the need for knowledge-based information. The hospital's services, resources, and systems for knowledge-based information are based on a thorough needs assessment, which addresses
- the needs of those who will use the information;
- accessibility and timeliness;
- links with the hospital's internal information systems; and
- links with external databases and information networks.

Standard IM.5
Transmission of data and information is timely and accurate.

Intent of IM.5
Internally and externally generated data and information are accurately transmitted to users. The integrity of data and information is maintained, and adequate communication exists between data users and suppliers. Specific attention is directed to the processes for ensuring accurate, timely, and complete verbal and written communication among care-givers and all others involved in the utilization of data. The timing of transmission is appropriate to the data's intended use.

Standard IM.7
The hospital defines, captures, analyzes, transforms, transmits, and reports patient-specific data and information related to care processes and outcomes.

Standard IM.7.1
The hospital initiates and maintains a medical record for every individual assessed or treated.

Standard IM.7.1.1
Only authorized individuals make entries in medical records.

Standard IM.7.1.2

The hospital determines how long medical record information is retained, based on law and regulation and the information used for patient care, legal, research, and educational purposes.

Standard IM.7.2

The medical record contains sufficient information to identify the patient, support the diagnosis, justify the treatment, document the course and results, and promote continuity of care among health care providers.

Intent of IM.7 Through IM.7.2

Information management processes provide for the use of patient-specific data and information to
- facilitate patient care;
- serve as a financial and legal record;
- aid in clinical research;
- support decision analysis; and
- guide professional and organizational performance improvement.

To facilitate consistency and continuity in patient care, specific data and information are required. Administrative and direct patient care providers produce and use this information for professional and organization improvement. Medical records contain sufficient information to
- identify the patient;
- support the diagnosis;
- justify the treatment;
- document the course and results; and
- facilitate continuity of care.

The environment in which patient-specific information is provided supports timely, accurate, secure, and confidential recording and use of patient-specific information. The system recalls historical patient data and is able to furnish data about current encounters. To facilitate consistency and continuity in patient care, the medical record contains very specific data and information, including
- the patient's name, address, date of birth, and the name of any legally authorized representative;

- the legal status of patients receiving mental health services;
- emergency care provided to the patient prior to arrival, if any;
- the record and findings of the patient's assessment;
- conclusions or impressions drawn from the medical history and physical examination;
- the diagnosis or diagnostic impression;
- the reasons for admission or treatment;
- the goals of treatment and the treatment plan;
- evidence of known advance directives;
- evidence of informed consent, when required by hospital policy;
- diagnostic and therapeutic orders, if any;
- all diagnostic and therapeutic procedures and test results;
- test results relevant to the management of the patient's condition;
- all operative and other invasive procedures performed, using acceptable disease and operative terminology that includes etiology, as appropriate;
- progress notes made by the medical staff and other authorized individuals;
- all reassessments and any revisions of the treatment plan;
- clinical observations;
- the patient's response to care;
- consultation reports;
- every medication ordered or prescribed for an inpatient;
- every medication dispensed to an ambulatory patient or an inpatient on discharge;
- every dose of medication administered and any adverse drug reaction;
- all relevant diagnoses established during the course of care;
- any referrals and communications made to external or internal care providers and to community agencies;
- conclusions at termination of hospitalization;
- discharge instructions to the patient and family; and

- clinical résumés and discharge summaries, or a final progress note or transfer summary.

A concise clinical résumés included in the medical record at discharge provides important information to other caregivers and facilitates continuity of care. For patients discharged to ambulatory (outpatient) care, the clinical résumé summarizes previous levels of care. The discharge summary contains the following information:

- The reason for hospitalization;
- Significant findings;
- Procedures performed and treatment rendered;
- The patient's condition at discharge; and
- Instructions to the patient and family, if any.

For newborns with uncomplicated deliveries, or for patients hospitalized for less than 48 hours with only minor problems, a progress note may be substituted for the clinical résumé. The medical staff defines what problems and interventions may be considered minor. The progress note, which may be handwritten, documents the patient's condition at discharge, discharge instructions, and required follow-up care.

When a patient is transferred within the same organization from one level of care to another (for example, from the hospital to residential care), and the caregivers change, a transfer summary may be substituted for the clinical résumé. A transfer summary briefly describes the patient's condition at time of transfer, and the reason for the transfer. When the caregivers remain the same, a progress note may suffice.

Standard IM.8
The hospital collects and aggregates data and information to support care and service delivery and operations.

Intent of IM.8
Certain types of data and information need to be accumulated over time to support the hospital's clinical and management functions. The hospital assesses its need for aggregated data and information and defines the types of required data and information. The information management function has the ability to collect and aggregate clinical and administrative data to support

- individual care and care delivery;
- decision making;
- management and operations;
- analysis of trends over time;
- performance comparisons over time within the hospital and with other hospitals;
- performance improvement; and
- reduction in risks to patients.

The hospital is able to aggregate the data and information requirements specified in this manual, as well as identified indicator data for performance measurement.

Standard IM.9
Knowledge-based information systems, resources, and services meet the hospital's needs.

Intent of IM.9
Appropriate knowledge-based information is acquired, assembled, and transmitted to users. Knowledge-based information management consists of systems, resources, and services to

- help health professionals acquire and maintain the knowledge and skills they need to maintain and improve competence;
- support clinical and management decision making;
- support performance improvement and activities to reduce risk to patients;
- provide needed information and education to individuals and families; and
- satisfy research-related needs.

Knowledge-based information refers to current authoritative print and nonprint information resources, including

- current periodicals, indexes, and abstracts in print or electronic format;

- other clinical and managerial literature;
- successful practices;
- practice guidelines;
- research data;
- recent editions of texts and other resources;
- satellite television services; and
- on-line computer-linked information services via the Internet.

All types of information do not have to be provided on site. A hospital is not required to have a library located in its facility. Services may be shared with hospitals or community resources as long as information is accessible to the hospital's staff in a timely manner.

INDEX